Quick and Easy Mediterranean Recipes:

100+ Recipes for Beginners to Live a Healthier Life with Taste.

TABLE OF CONTENTS

INTRODUCTION

For decades now, researchers have consistently found that people who follow the Mediterranean Diet pattern generally have less chronic disease, along with reductions in blood pressure, blood lipids, and weight. The Mediterranean Diet also helps reduce long-term blood sugar levels, according to a 2013 study published in the American Journal of Clinical Nutrition. All of these overwhelmingly positive results have led doctors, dietitians, diabetes educators, and many health care professionals to recommend the Mediterranean Diet to their patients year after year. In fact, it's one of only three eating patterns recommended in the current edition of Dietary Guidelines for Americans.

The many health benefits tied to this eating lifestyle include reduced risk of:

Alzheimer's disease: As we age, our brains shrink. In several studies, including one published in Neurology in 2017, researchers found that people who eat according to the Mediterranean Diet generally maintain a bigger brain size than those who don't eat this way. Some doctors speculate that having a larger brain may help lower the risk of brain diseases, including dementia and Alzheimer's.

Arthritis: In a handful of studies, researchers have found associations between eating the Mediterranean Diet and a reduction in pain caused by osteoarthritis and rheumatoid arthritis. Specific symptom-relieving foods include extra-virgin olive oil and fiber-rich whole grains, according to a 2013 study in the Journal of Nutritional Biochemistry.

Asthma: In both Mediterranean and non-Mediterranean countries, scientists have found the Mediterranean Diet seems to have a protective effect against asthma and wheezing in children, according to a 2017 study in Public Health Nutrition. In some studies, this association was also seen in the babies of mothers eating the Mediterranean Diet.

Cancer: There is a strong consensus among health care professionals that following the Mediterranean Diet is linked to reduced overall cancer rates. Cancer-lowering associations are even stronger for digestive tract cancers, as reported in a 2017 study in Cancer Genomics and Proteomics.

Cardiovascular disease: Most health care professionals agree that the Mediterranean Diet lowers the danger of heart disease, an association mentioned in Dietary Guidelines for Americans.

Diabetes: Nutrition researchers have repeatedly found associations between lower rates of type 2 diabetes and this diet. In some of the most compelling trials, published in 2018 in Nutrition & Diabetes, researchers compared a low-fat diet to the much higher-fat Mediterranean Diet and found that, among other health indicators, diabetes rates were lower in people eating the Mediterranean Diet.

High blood pressure: The healthy fats found in the Mediterranean Diet are probably one of the keys to the lower blood pressure rates found in people following this eating pattern. These healthier fats include the monounsaturated fats found in olive oil and some nuts and the omega-3 fats found in most fish.

High cholesterol: It's likely the Mediterranean Diet can lower the danger of heart disease partially since individuals eating this method have lower levels of LDL blood cholesterol. LDLs are the "bad" cholesterol, which are more apt to build up deposits in your arteries.

In January 2018, after reviewing 40 different diet plans, U.S. News & World Report magazine and a panel of health experts ranked the Mediterranean Diet as a Best Diet Overall (tied with the DASH diet), as well as the easiest diet plan to follow.

BREAKFAST RECIPES

1. Raspberry Vanilla Smoothie

Preparation Time: 5 minutes

Cooking Time: 5 minutes

Servings: 2 cups

INGREDIENTS:

- 1 cup frozen raspberries
- 6-ounce container of vanilla Greek yogurt
- ½ cup of unsweetened vanilla almond milk

DIRECTIONS:

1. Take all of your ingredients and place them in a blender. Process until smooth and liquified.

NUTRITION: Calories: 155 Protein: 7 g Fat: 2 g Carbohydrates: 30 g

2. Blueberry Banana Protein Smoothie

Preparation Time: 5 minutes

Cooking Time: 5 minutes

Servings: 1

INGREDIENTS:

- ½ cup frozen and unsweetened blueberries
- ½ banana slices up
- ¾ cup plain nonfat Greek yogurt

- ¾ cup unsweetened vanilla almond milk
- 2 cups of ice cubes

DIRECTIONS:

1. Add all of the ingredients into a blender. Blend until smooth.

NUTRITION: Calories: 230 Protein: 19.1 g Fat: 2.6 g Carbohydrates: 32.9 g

3. Chocolate Banana Smoothie

Preparation Time: 5 minutes

Cooking Time: 0 minutes

Servings: 2

INGREDIENTS:

- 2 bananas, peeled
- 1 cup unsweetened almond milk, or skim milk
- 1 cup crushed ice
- 3 tablespoons unsweetened cocoa powder
- 3 tablespoons honey

DIRECTIONS:

1. In a blender, combine the bananas, almond milk, ice, cocoa powder, and honey. Blend until smooth.

NUTRITION: Calories: 219 Protein: 2g Carbohydrates: 57g Fat: 2g

4. Moroccan Avocado Smoothie

Preparation Time: 5 minutes

Cooking Time: 0 minutes

Servings: 4

INGREDIENTS:

- 1 ripe avocado, peeled and pitted
- 1 overripe banana
- 1 cup almond milk, unsweetened
- 1 cup of ice

DIRECTIONS:

1. Place the avocado, banana, milk, and ice into your blender. Blend until smooth with no pieces of avocado remaining.

NUTRITION: Calories: 100 Protein: 1 g Fat: 6 g Carbohydrates: 11 g

5. Mango Pear Smoothie

Preparation Time: 5 minutes

Cooking Time: 0 minute

Servings: 1

INGREDIENTS:

- 2 ice cubes
- ½ cup Greek yogurt, plain
- ½ mango, peeled, pitted & chopped
- 1 cup kale, chopped
- 1 pear, ripe, cored & chopped

DIRECTIONS:

1. Take all ingredients and place them in your blender. Blend together until thick and smooth. Serve.

NUTRITION: Calories 350 Protein 40g Fats 12g Carbohydrates: 11 g

6. Mediterranean Smoothie

Preparation Time: 5 minutes

Cooking Time: 5 minutes

Servings: 2

INGREDIENTS:

- 2 cups of baby spinach
- 1 teaspoon fresh ginger root
- 1 frozen banana, pre-sliced
- 1 small mango
- ½ cup beet juice
- ½ cup of skim milk
- 4-6 ice cubes

DIRECTIONS:

1. Take all ingredients and place them in your blender. Blend together until thick and smooth. Serve.

NUTRITION: Calories: 168 Protein: 4 g Fat: 1 g Carbohydrates: 39 g

7. Fruit Smoothie

Preparation Time: 5 minutes

Cooking Time: 0 minutes

Servings: 2

INGREDIENTS:

- 2 cups blueberries (or any fresh or frozen fruit, cut into pieces if the fruit is large)

- 2 cups unsweetened almond milk

- 1 cup crushed ice

- ½ teaspoon ground ginger (or other dried ground spice such as turmeric, cinnamon, or nutmeg)

DIRECTIONS:

1. In a blender, combine the blueberries, almond milk, ice, and ginger. Blend until smooth.

NUTRITION: Calories: 125 Protein: 2g Carbohydrates: 23g Fat: 4g

8. Strawberry-Rhubarb Smoothie

Preparation Time: 5 minutes

Cooking Time: 3 minutes

Servings: 1

INGREDIENTS:

- 1 rhubarb stalk, chopped

- 1 cup sliced fresh strawberries

- ½ cup plain Greek yogurt

- 2 tablespoons honey

- Pinch ground cinnamon

- 3 ice cubes

DIRECTIONS:

1. Place a small saucepan filled with water over high heat and bring to a boil. Add the rhubarb and boil for 3 minutes. Drain and transfer the rhubarb to a blender.

2. Add the strawberries, yogurt, honey, and cinnamon and pulse the mixture until it is smooth. Add the ice and blend until thick, with no ice lumps remaining. Pour the smoothie into a glass and enjoy cold.

NUTRITION: Calories: 295 Fat: 8g Carbohydrates: 56g Protein: 6g

9. Chia-Pomegranate Smoothie

Preparation Time: 5 minutes

Cooking Time: 0 minutes

Servings: 2

INGREDIENTS:

- 1 cup pure pomegranate juice (no sugar added)
- 1 cup frozen berries
- 1 cup coarsely chopped kale
- 2 tablespoons chia seeds
- 3 Medjool dates, pitted and coarsely chopped
- Pinch ground cinnamon

DIRECTIONS:

1. In a blender, combine the pomegranate juice, berries, kale, chia seeds, dates, and cinnamon and pulse until smooth. Pour into glasses and serve.

NUTRITION: Calories: 275 Fat: 5g Carbohydrates: 59g Protein: 5g

RICE, BEAN, AND GRAIN

RECIPES

10. Quinoa and Chickpea Vegetable Bowls

Preparation time: 15 minutes

Cooking time: 15 minutes

Servings: 4

INGREDIENTS:

- 1 cup red dry quinoa, rinsed and drained
- 2 cups low-sodium vegetable soup
- 2 cups fresh spinach
- 2 cups finely shredded red cabbage
- 1 (15-ounce / 425-g) can chickpeas, drained and rinsed
- 1 ripe avocado, thinly sliced
- 1 cup shredded carrots
- 1 red bell pepper, thinly sliced
- 4 tablespoons Mango Sauce
- ½ cup fresh cilantro, chopped
- Mango Sauce:
- 1 mango, diced
- ¼ cup fresh lime juice

- ½ teaspoon ground turmeric
- 1 teaspoon finely minced fresh ginger
- ¼ teaspoon sea salt
- Pinch of ground red pepper
- 1 teaspoon pure maple syrup
- 2 tablespoons extra-virgin olive oil

DIRECTIONS:

1. Pour the quinoa and vegetable soup in a saucepan. Bring to a boil. Reduce the heat to low. Cover and cook for 15 minutes or until tender. Fluffy with a fork.

2. Meanwhile, combine the ingredients for the mango sauce in a food processor. Pulse until smooth.

3. Divide the quinoa, spinach, and cabbage into 4 serving bowls, then top with chickpeas, avocado, carrots, and bell pepper.

4. Dress them with the mango sauce and spread with cilantro. Serve immediately.

NUTRITION: Calories: 366 Fat: 11.1g Protein: 15.5g Carbs: 55.6g

11. Ritzy Veggie Chili

Preparation time: 15 minutes

Cooking time: 5 hours

Servings: 4

INGREDIENTS:

- 1 (28-ounce / 794-g) can chopped tomatoes, with the juice
- 1 (15-ounce / 425-g) can black beans, drained and rinsed

- 1 (15-ounce / 425-g) can redly beans, drained and rinsed
- 1 medium green bell pepper, chopped
- 1 yellow onion, chopped
- 1 tablespoon onion powder
- 1 teaspoon paprika
- 1 teaspoon cayenne pepper
- 1 teaspoon garlic powder
- ½ teaspoon sea salt
- ½ teaspoon ground black pepper
- 1 tablespoon olive oil
- 1 large hass avocado, pitted, peeled, and chopped, for garnish

DIRECTIONS:

1. Combine all the ingredients, except for the avocado, in the slow cooker. Stir to mix well.
2. Put the slow cooker lid on and cook on high for 5 hours or until the vegetables are tender and the mixture has a thick consistency.
3. Pour the chili in a large serving bowl. Allow to cool for 30 minutes, then spread with chopped avocado and serve.

NUTRITION: Calories: 633 Fat: 16.3g Protein: 31.7g Carbs: 97.0g

12. Spicy Italian Bean Balls with Marinara

Preparation time: 15 minutes

Cooking time: 30 minutes

Servings: 2-4

INGREDIENTS:

- Bean Balls:
- 1 tablespoon extra-virgin olive oil
- ½ yellow onion, minced
- 1 teaspoon fennel seeds
- 2 teaspoons dried oregano
- ½ teaspoon crushed red pepper flakes
- 1 teaspoon garlic powder
- 1 (15-ounce / 425-g) can white beans (cannellini or navy), drained and rinsed
- ½ cup whole-grain bread crumbs
- Sea salt and ground black pepper, to taste
- Marinara:
- 1 tablespoon extra-virgin olive oil
- 3 garlic cloves, minced
- Handful basil leaves
- 1 (28-ounce / 794-g) can chopped tomatoes with juice reserved
- Sea salt, to taste

DIRECTIONS:

1. Preheat the oven to 350°F (180°C). Line a baking sheet with parchment paper. Heat the olive oil in a nonstick skillet over medium heat until shimmering.

2. Add the onion and sauté for 5 minutes or until translucent. Sprinkle with fennel seeds, oregano, red pepper flakes, and garlic powder, then cook for 1 minute or until aromatic.

3. Pour the sautéed mixture in a food processor and add the beans and bread crumbs. Sprinkle with salt and ground black pepper, then pulse to combine well and the mixture holds together.

4. Shape the mixture into balls with a 2-ounce (57-g) cookie scoop, then arrange the balls on the baking sheet.

5. Bake in the preheated oven for 30 minutes or until lightly browned. Flip the balls halfway through the cooking time.

6. While baking the bean balls, heat the olive oil in a saucepan over medium-high heat until shimmering. Add the garlic and basil and sauté for 2 minutes or until fragrant.

7. Fold in the tomatoes and juice. Bring to a boil. Reduce the heat to low. Put the lid on and simmer for 15 minutes. Sprinkle with salt.

8. Transfer the bean balls on a large plate and baste with marinara before serving.

NUTRITION: Calories: 351 Fat: 16.4g Protein: 11.5g Carbs: 42.9g

13. Baked Rolled Oat with Pears and Pecans

Preparation time: 15 minutes

Cooking time: 30 minutes

Servings: 6

INGREDIENTS:

- 2 tablespoons coconut oil, melted, plus more for greasing the pan
- 3 ripe pears, cored and diced

- 2 cups unsweetened almond milk
- 1 tablespoon pure vanilla extract
- ¼ cup pure maple syrup
- 2 cups gluten-free rolled oats
- ½ cup raisins
- ¾ cup chopped pecans
- ¼ teaspoon ground nutmeg
- 1 teaspoon ground cinnamon
- ½ teaspoon ground ginger
- ¼ teaspoon sea salt

DIRECTIONS:

1. Preheat the oven to 350°F (180°C). Grease a baking dish with melted coconut oil, then spread the pears in a single layer on the baking dish evenly.

2. Combine the almond milk, vanilla extract, maple syrup, and coconut oil in a bowl. Stir to mix well.

3. Combine the remaining ingredients in a separate large bowl. Stir to mix well. Fold the almond milk mixture in the bowl, then pour the mixture over the pears.

4. Place the baking dish in the preheated oven and bake for 30 minutes or until lightly browned and set. Serve immediately.

NUTRITION: Calories: 479 Fat: 34.9g Protein: 8.8g Carbs: 50.1g

14. Brown Rice Pilaf with Pistachios and Raisins

Preparation time: 15 minutes

Cooking time: 15 minutes

Servings: 6

INGREDIENTS:

- 1 tablespoon extra-virgin olive oil
- 1 cup chopped onion
- ½ cup shredded carrot
- ½ teaspoon ground cinnamon
- 1 teaspoon ground cumin
- 2 cups brown rice
- 1¾ cups pure orange juice
- ¼ cup water
- ½ cup shelled pistachios
- 1 cup golden raisins
- ½ cup chopped fresh chives

DIRECTIONS:

1. Heat the olive oil in a saucepan over medium-high heat until shimmering. Add the onion and sauté for 5 minutes or until translucent.

2. Add the carrots, cinnamon, and cumin, then sauté for 1 minutes or until aromatic.

3. Pour int the brown rice, orange juice, and water. Bring to a boil. Reduce the heat to medium-low and simmer for 7 minutes or until the liquid is almost absorbed.

4. Transfer the rice mixture in a large serving bowl, then spread with pistachios, raisins, and chives. Serve immediately.

NUTRITION: Calories: 264 Fat: 7.1g Protein: 5.2g Carbs: 48.9g

15. Cherry, Apricot, and Pecan Brown Rice Bowl

Preparation time: 15 minutes

Cooking time: 1 hour & 1 minute

Servings: 2

INGREDIENTS:

- 2 tablespoons olive oil
- 2 green onions, sliced
- ½ cup brown rice
- 1 cup low -sodium chicken stock
- 2 tablespoons dried cherries
- 4 dried apricots, chopped
- 2 tablespoons pecans, toasted and chopped
- Sea salt and freshly ground pepper, to taste

DIRECTIONS:

1. Heat the olive oil in a medium saucepan over medium-high heat until shimmering. Add the green onions and sauté for 1 minutes or until fragrant.

2. Add the rice. Stir to mix well, then pour in the chicken stock. Bring to a boil. Reduce the heat to low. Cover and simmer for 50 minutes or until the brown rice is soft.

3. Add the cherries, apricots, and pecans, and simmer for 10 more minutes or until the fruits are tender.

4. Pour them in a large serving bowl. Fluff with a fork. Sprinkle with sea salt and freshly ground pepper. Serve immediately.

NUTRITION: Calories: 451 Fat: 25.9g Protein: 8.2g Carbs: 50.4g

16. Curry Apple Couscous with Leeks and Pecans

Preparation time: 15 minutes

Cooking time: 8 minutes

Servings: 4

INGREDIENTS:

- 2 teaspoons extra-virgin olive oil
- 2 leeks, white parts only, sliced
- 1 apple, diced
- 2 cups cooked couscous
- 2 tablespoons curry powder
- ½ cup chopped pecans

DIRECTIONS:

1. Heat the olive oil in a skillet over medium heat until shimmering. Add the leeks and sauté for 5 minutes or until soft.

2. Add the diced apple and cook for 3 more minutes until tender. Add the couscous and curry powder. Stir to combine. Transfer them in a large serving bowl, then mix in the pecans and serve.

NUTRITION: Calories: 254 Fat: 11.9g Protein: 5.4g Carbs: 34.3g

17. Lebanese Flavor Broken Thin Noodles

Preparation time: 15 minutes

Cooking time: 25 minutes

Servings: 6

INGREDIENTS:

- 1 tablespoon extra-virgin olive oil
- 1 (3-ounce / 85-g) cup vermicelli, broken into 1- to 1½-inch pieces
- 3 cups shredded cabbage
- 1 cup brown rice
- 3 cups low-sodium vegetable soup
- ½ cup water
- 2 garlic cloves, mashed
- ¼ teaspoon sea salt
- 1/8 teaspoon crushed red pepper flakes
- ½ cup coarsely chopped cilantro
- Fresh lemon slices, for serving

DIRECTIONS:

1. Heat the olive oil in a saucepan over medium-high heat until shimmering. Add the vermicelli and sauté for 3 minutes or until

toasted. Add the cabbage and sauté for 4 minutes or until tender.

2. Pour in the brown rice, vegetable soup, and water. Add the garlic and sprinkle with salt and red pepper flakes.

3. Bring to a boil over high heat. Reduce the heat to medium low. Put the lid on and simmer for another 10 minutes. Turn off the heat, then let sit for 5 minutes without opening the lid.

4. Pour them on a large serving platter and spread with cilantro. Squeeze the lemon slices over and serve warm.

NUTRITION: Calories: 127 Fat: 3.1g Protein: 4.2g Carbs: 22.9g

18. Lemony Farro and Avocado Bowl

Preparation time: 15 minutes

Cooking time: 25 minutes

Servings: 4

INGREDIENTS:

- 1 tablespoon plus 2 teaspoons extra-virgin olive oil, divided
- ½ medium onion, chopped
- 1 carrot, shredded
- 2 garlic cloves, minced
- 1 (6-ounce / 170-g) cup pearled farro
- 2 cups low-sodium vegetable soup
- 2 avocados, peeled, pitted, and sliced
- Zest and juice of 1 small lemon
- ¼ teaspoon sea salt

DIRECTIONS:

1. Heat 1 tablespoon of olive oil in a saucepan over medium-high heat until shimmering. Add the onion and sauté for 5 minutes or until translucent. Add the carrot and garlic and sauté for 1 minute or until fragrant.

2. Add the farro and pour in the vegetable soup. Bring to a boil over high heat. Reduce the heat to low. Put the lid on and simmer for 20 minutes or until the farro is al dente.

3. Transfer the farro in a large serving bowl, then fold in the avocado slices. Sprinkle with lemon zest and salt, then drizzle with lemon juice and 2 teaspoons of olive oil. Stir to mix well and serve immediately.

NUTRITION: Calories: 210 Fat: 11.1g Protein: 4.2g Carbs: 27.9g

19. Rice and Blueberry Stuffed Sweet Potatoes

Preparation time: 15 minutes

Cooking time: 20 minutes

Servings: 4

INGREDIENTS:

- 2 cups cooked wild rice
- ½ cup dried blueberries
- ½ cup chopped hazelnuts
- ½ cup shredded Swiss chard
- 1 teaspoon chopped fresh thyme

- 1 scallion, white and green parts, peeled and thinly sliced

- Sea salt and freshly ground black pepper, to taste

- 4 sweet potatoes, baked in the skin until tender

DIRECTIONS:

1. Preheat the oven to 400°F (205°C). Combine all the ingredients, except for the sweet potatoes, in a large bowl. Stir to mix well.

2. Cut the top third of the sweet potato off length wire, then scoop most of the sweet potato flesh out. Fill the potato with the wild rice mixture, then set the sweet potato on a greased baking sheet.

3. Bake in the preheated oven for 20 minutes or until the sweet potato skin is lightly charred. Serve immediately.

NUTRITION: Calories: 393 Fat: 7.1g Protein: 10.2g Carbs: 76.9g

SOUP RECIPES

20. Artichoke Soup

Preparation Time: 15 minutes

Cooking Time: 15 minutes

Servings: 2

INGREDIENTS:

- pound capital of Israel artichokes
- tablespoons further virgin olive oil
- massive onion, thinly sliced
- 2 pound potatoes, bare-assed and diced
- 5 cups of water
- a grating of nutmeg salt
- Freshly ground black pepper
- tablespoons Petroselinum crispum, finely chopped

DIRECTIONS

1. Scrub the Jerusalem artichokes and peel them thinly, cutting away any stringy roots or tips. Heat the vegetable oil

2. In an exceedingly massive cooking pan and cook the onion over moderate heat till it's clear.

3. Add the capital of Israel artichokes and potatoes and simmer for five minutes, stirring once or double

4. Therefore, the vegetables cook equally. Add the water and produce to a boil.

5. Cowl and simmer for twenty minutes or till the vegetables are tender.

6. You should force it thru a sieve or puree in a totally liquidizer. Come back to the pan and warmth totally.

7. Finally, you should Season it with nutmeg, salt, & black pepper. Serve hot, fancy with parsley.

NUTRITION: Calories: 123, Fats: 3g, Dietary Fiber: 5g, Carbohydrates: 19g, Protein: 5g

21. Dalmatian Potato Soup

Preparation Time: 15 minutes
Cooking Time: 15 minutes
Servings: 2
INGREDIENTS:

- pound potatoes
- tablespoons further virgin olive oil
- massive onion, chopped
- ripe plum tomatoes, peeled, seeded, and chopped
- bay leaf
- cups water
- tablespoons butter
- tablespoons Petroselinum crispum, finely chopped
- tablespoons contemporary basil leaves, cut salt

- Freshly ground black pepper

DIRECTIONS

1. Peel and dice the potatoes heat the vegetable oil.
2. In an exceedingly large pot and cook the onion over a moderate heat till it's clear.
3. Add the potatoes, tomatoes, bay leaf, and water, and produce to a boil. Cover and simmer for half-hour.
4. Remove the herb. Force the soup through a sieve or puree in an exceedingly liquidizer.
5. Come back to the pot and warmth totally. Add the butter, parsley, and basil, and after that you should Season it with salt & black pepper.
6. Simmer for five minutes and serve hot.

NUTRITION: Calories: 123, Fats: 3g, Dietary Fiber: 5g, Carbohydrates: 19g, Protein: 5g

22. Pumpkin Soup with Rice and Spinach

Preparation Time: 15 minutes

Cooking Time: 15 minutes

Servings: 2

INGREDIENTS:

- 3 small pumpkins, concerning one pound
- 2 tablespoons extra virgin olive oil
- medium onion, chopped
- leek, white half only
- medium potatoes, bare-assed and diced

- cups vegetable stock or water
- cups milk
- 1 bay leaf
- A sprig of thyme
- A grating of nutmeg
- Salt
- Freshly ground black pepper
- cup Arborio rice
- 2-pound spinach
- tablespoons butter
- Freshly grated Parmesan cheese

DIRECTIONS

1. Slice the pumpkin. stop the skin and take away the seeds and pith.
2. Dice the flesh into little items. Heat the vegetable oil in an exceedingly massive cooking pan and cook the onion and leek over a moderate heat till they're softened.
3. Add the pumpkin, potatoes, stock or water, milk, and herbs and produce to a boil. cowl and simmer for 30 minutes or till the vegetables are tender. Season with nutmeg, salt, and black pepper.
4. Remove the herb and thyme. You should force it via a sieve or puree in an exceedingly liquidizer.
5. Return to the pot, adding a touch a lot of water if the soup is simply too thick. Rouse a boil.

6. Add the rice and cook for twenty a lot of minutes or till the rice is tender but still firm.

7. Meanwhile, wash the spinach carefully and cook in an exceedingly lined pan over a moderate heat for five minutes or till it is simply tender. Drain well and chop coarsely.

8. Melt 1/2 the butter in an exceedingly cooking pan and cook the spinach over a delicate heat for three or four minutes.

9. Augment the soup. Stir within the remaining butter and serve hot with cheese on the facet.

NUTRITION: Calories: 123, Fats: 3g, Dietary Fiber: 5g, Carbohydrates: 19g, Protein: 5g

23. Nettle Soup

Preparation Time: 15 minutes
Cooking Time: 15 minutes
Servings: 2
INGREDIENTS:

- 6 ounces nettles
- 3 tablespoons further virgin olive oil
- 2 medium onions, sliced
- pound potatoes, bare-assed and diced
- 5 cups water
- cup crème fraiche
- Salt
- Freshly ground black pepper

DIRECTIONS

1. Wash the nettles fastidiously and put aside.

2. Heat the olive oil in an exceedingly massive cooking pan and cook the onions over a moderate heat for five minutes.

3. Add the nettles, potatoes, and water, and produce to a boil.

4. Cover and simmer for half-hour. Force through a sieve or puree in an exceedingly liquidizer.

5. Return to the cooking pan and warmth totally.

6. Stir within the crème fraiche and after that you should Season it with salt & black pepper.

NUTRITION: 195 Calories 9.6g Fat 7.6g Protein

24. Wild Mushroom Soup

Preparation Time: 15 minutes

Cooking Time: 15 minutes

Servings: 2

INGREDIENTS:

- pound mixed wild mushrooms
- 4 tablespoons further virgin olive oil
- Spanish onion, chopped
- ripe plum tomatoes, peeled, seeded, and chopped
- 5 cups vegetable broth or water
- Salt
- Freshly ground black pepper
- FOR THE PICADA:

- 15 blanched almonds
- slice white bread concerning one in. thick (crust removed)
- 1-2 tablespoons further virgin olive oil
- garlic cloves, crushed
- Pinch of saffron powder

DIRECTIONS

1. To build the soup, wash the mushrooms fastidiously and wipe dry.

2. Cut them into three or four items consistent with their size and heat the vegetable oil

3. In an exceedingly massive pan and cook the onion over a delicate heat for concerning ten minutes or till it starts to show golden.

4. Add the tomatoes and still cook till any liquid is gaseous and also the tomatoes are reduced to a pulp.

5. Stir within the mushrooms.

6. Cowl and simmer for quarter-hour, stirring from time to time therefore the mushrooms cook equally.

7. You should add the broth & convey to a boil. Simmer, uncovered, for twenty minutes. After that you should Season it with salt & black pepper.

8. To build the picada, toast the almonds in an exceedingly 350°F kitchen appliance until they're golden chop coarsely.

9. Heat one or a pair of tablespoons vegetable oil in an exceedingly small cooking pan.

10. And fry the bread till it's golden on each side drain on a paper towel and withdraw little items or Crush or grind the almonds, deep-fried bread, garlic, and saffron with a mortar and pestle

11. In an exceedingly kitchen appliance, till all the ingredients type a sleek, thick paste.

12. Mix with a tablespoon or 2 of the soup into the picada, then stir the mixture into the soup.

13. Place a slice of bread on the lowest of 4 man or woman soup bowls. Pour the new soup over the bread and serve.

NUTRITION: 195 Calories 9.6g Fat 7.6g Protein

25. Tomato and Alimentary Paste Soup

Preparation Time: 15 minutes

Cooking Time: 15 minutes

Servings: 2

INGREDIENTS:

- 3 tablespoons further virgin olive oil
- massive onion, chopped
- garlic cloves, finely chopped
- 1-2 red chili peppers, cored, seeded, and finely chopped
- cup canned plum tomatoes, forced through a sieve or pureed in a food processor
- bunch Petroselinum crispum, finely chopped
- 6 cups water
- ounces fine alimentary paste or (angel hair)

- Salt

DIRECTIONS

1. Heat the vegetable oil in an exceedingly massive pot and cook the onion over moderate heat till it's softened.

2. Add the garlic and chili peppers and cook for two a lot of minutes.

3. Add the tomato puree and parsley and cook for a further five minutes.

4. Pour within the water and produce to a boil. Simmer for ten minutes.

5. Increase the warmth. Once the soup is boiling, come by the alimentary paste and cook till it's tender however still firm.

6. Finally, you need to Season it with salt and serve hot.

NUTRITION: Calories: 123, Fats: 3g, Dietary Fiber: 5g, Carbohydrates: 19g, Protein: 5g

26. Sorrel Soup

Preparation Time: 15 minutes

Cooking Time: 15 minutes

Servings: 2

INGREDIENTS:

- 1-pound sorrel
- 3 tablespoons butter
- 3 tablespoons flour
- 5 cups quandary (or .05 water and half milk)
- A grating of nutmeg

- Salt
- Freshly ground black pepper

DIRECTIONS

1. Wash the sorrel fastidiously and take away the stalks and larger ribs.

2. Heat the butter in an exceedingly massive cooking pan and add the sorrel.

3. Cover and cook over a delicate heat till the sorrel has softened into a puree.

4. Stir within the flour and cook for two minutes.

5. Gradually add the new water, stirring perpetually, till the soup is slightly thickened.

6. Simmer for twenty minutes. Finally, you must season it with nutmeg, salt, and black pepper.

27. Summer Vegetable Soup

Preparation Time: 15 minutes

Cooking Time: 15 minutes

Servings: 2

INGREDIENTS:

- medium eggplant (about ~ pound)
- pound zucchini
- red, green, or yellow bell peppers
- cup further virgin olive oil
- massive onion, thinly sliced

- celery stalks, diced

- pound waxy potatoes, peeled and diced

- 2-pound ripe plum tomatoes, peeled, seeded, and chopped

- cups water

- 2 tablespoons torn basil leaves

- Salt

- Freshly ground black pepper

- Freshly grated pecorino or Parmesan cheese

DIRECTIONS

1. Peel and dice the eggplant. Trim the ends of the zucchini and withdraw rounds.

2. Cut the peppers into quarters and take away the cores and seeds. withdraw skinny strips and heat the vegetable oil

3. In an exceedingly massive pot and cook the onion, celery, and potatoes over a coffee heat for ten minutes

4. Stirring from time to time therefore the vegetables cook equally.

5. Add the eggplant, zucchini, and peppers, cover, and cook for an additional ten minutes.

6. Add the tomatoes and cook, uncovered, for 10 more minutes.

7. Pour within the water and produce to a boil.

8. Cowl and simmer for fifteen to 20 minutes or till the vegetables are tender.

9. The soup ought to be terribly thick, almost a stew.

10. Add the basil and simmer for two or three minutes.

11. After that you should Season it with salt & black pepper. Serve hot with cheese on the facet.

NUTRITION: Calories: 123, Fats: 3g, Dietary Fiber: 5g, Carbohydrates: 19g, Protein: 5g

28. Tuscan Black Cabbage Soup

Preparation Time: 15 minutes
Cooking Time: 15 minutes
Servings: 2
INGREDIENTS:

- pound Tuscan black cabbage
- tablespoons further virgin olive oil
- large onion, thinly sliced
- celery stalk, thinly sliced
- carrot, diced
- medium potato, bare-assed and diced
- 5 cups vegetable broth or water
- Salt
- Freshly ground black pepper
- slices wheaten bread
- garlic cloves, peeled, and cut in half
- Freshly grated Parmesan cheese

DIRECTIONS

1. Wash the cabbage and take away the stalks. Withdraw skinny strips and heat the vegetable oil

2. in an exceedingly massive pot and cook the onion, celery, carrot, and potato for three minutes.

3. Add the cabbage and broth and bring to a boil cowl and simmer for one hour and you should After that you should Season it with salt & black pepper.

4. Meanwhile place the slices of bread on a baking receptacle and toast

5. In an exceedingly preheated 375 ·p kitchen appliance till they're golden.

6. Take away from the kitchen appliance and rub every slice with garlic.

7. Place the slices of bread into individual soup bowls and pour the new soup over them.

8. Serve at once with cheese on the facet.

NUTRITION: Calories: 123, Fats: 3g, Dietary Fiber: 5g, Carbohydrates: 19g, Protein: 5g

29. Potato Leek Soup

Preparation Time: 10 minutes

Cooking Time: 20 minutes

Servings: 5

INGREDIENTS:

- 4 tablespoons of olive oil
- 3 leeks
- 3 cups of onions, diced
- 1 lb. of potatoes, diced
- 4 garlic cloves, chopped
- 1 tablespoon of thyme

- 6 cups of veggie stock
- ½ teaspoon of pepper
- 1 teaspoon of salt
- ½ cup of plant-based sour cream
- 2 tablespoons of chives, for garnishing

DIRECTIONS

1. Cut the leeks in half-length. Slice them into ¼-inch rounds.
2. Heat oil over medium heat in a pot or oven.
3. Add the leeks and sauté for 8 minutes.
4. Add the garlic. Sauté for 3 minutes more.
5. Add the thyme, potatoes, and stock. Boil. Turn the heat to a simmer for 20 minutes. Your potatoes should be tender.
6. Add the pepper and salt.
7. Blend in batches to make it very silky and smooth.
8. Return your soup to the pot. Simmer over low heat.
9. Stir the sour cream in. Serve with the chives.

NUTRITION: Calories 224 Carbohydrates 31g Cholesterol 10mg Fat 13g Protein 4g Sugar 4g Fiber 4g Sodium 337mg

30. Lentil Beet Soup

Preparation Time: 10 minutes

Cooking Time: 30 minutes

Servings: 2

INGREDIENTS:

- 1 shallot, chopped

- 2 teaspoons of olive oil

- 3 cloves of garlic, chopped

- 4 cups of water

- ½ cup of dry whole lentils

- 2 teaspoons of cumin

- 1 teaspoon of salt

- 1 lemon

- 2-3 cups of beets, grated

- Cilantro or parsley for garnishing

DIRECTIONS

1. Heat oil over medium heat in a pot. Sauté the shallot for 2 minutes.

2. Add the garlic. Sauté for 2 minutes more.

3. Add the beets, lentils, water, cumin, and salt. Cook for half an hour.

4. Squeeze the juice of one lemon when your lentils are tender.

5. Divide among two bowls. Top with the dill and grated beets.

NUTRITION: Calories 329 Carbohydrates 53g Cholesterol 0mg Fat 9g Protein 16g Sugar 13g Fiber 11g Sodium 308mg

MAIN RECIPES: MEAT

31. Grilled Steak, Mushroom, and Onion Kebabs

Preparation Time: 10 minutes

Cooking Time: 10 minutes

Servings: 2

INGREDIENTS:

- Boneless top sirloin steak, 1 lb.
- White button mushrooms, 8 oz.
- Medium red onion, 1.
- Peeled garlic cloves, 4.
- Rosemary sprigs, 2.
- Extra-virgin olive oil, 2 tbsp.
- Black pepper, ¼ tsp.
- Red wine vinegar, 2 tbsp.
- Sea salt, ¼ tsp.

DIRECTIONS:

1. Soak 12 (10-inch) wooden skewers in water. Spray the cold grill with nonstick cooking spray, and heat the grill to medium-high.
2. Cut a piece of aluminum foil into a 10-inch square. Place the garlic and rosemary sprigs in the center, drizzle with 1 tablespoon of oil, and wrap tightly to form a foil packet.

3. Arrange it on the grill, and seal the grill cover.

4. Cut the steak into 1-inch cubes. Thread the beef onto the wet skewers, alternating with whole mushrooms and onion wedges. Spray the kebabs thoroughly with nonstick cooking spray, and sprinkle with pepper.

5. Cook the kebabs on the covered grill for 5 minutes.

6. Flip and grill for 5 more minutes while covered.

7. Unwrap foil packets with garlic and rosemary sprigs and put them into a small bowl.

8. Carefully strip the rosemary sprigs of their leaves into the bowl and pour in any accumulated juices and oil from the foil packet.

9. Mix in the remaining 1 tablespoon of oil and the vinegar and salt.

10. Mash the garlic with a fork, and mix all ingredients in the bowl together. Pour over the finished steak kebabs and serve.

NUTRITION: Calories: 410, Protein: 36 g, Carbohydrates: 12 g, Fat: 14 g

32. Turkey Meatballs

Preparation Time: 10 minutes

Cooking Time: 25 minutes

Servings: 2

INGREDIENTS:

- Diced yellow onion, ¼
- Diced artichoke hearts, 14 oz.
- Ground turkey, 1 lb.

- Dried parsley, 1 tsp.

- Oil, 1 tsp.

- Chopped basil, 4 tbsp.

- Pepper and salt, to taste.

DIRECTIONS:

1. Grease the baking sheet and preheat the oven to 350^0 F.

2. On medium heat, place a nonstick medium saucepan, sauté artichoke hearts, and diced onions for 5 minutes or until onions are soft.

3. Meanwhile, in a big bowl, mix parsley, basil and ground turkey with hands. Season to taste.

4. Once onion mixture has cooled, add into the bowl and mix thoroughly.

5. With an ice cream scooper, scoop ground turkey and form balls.

6. Place on a prepared cooking sheet, pop in the oven and bake until cooked around 15-20 minutes.

7. Remove from pan, serve and enjoy

NUTRITION: Calories: 283, Protein: 12 g, Carbohydrates: 30 g, Fat: 12 g

33. Chicken Marsala

Preparation Time: 10 minutes

Cooking Time: 45 minutes

Servings: 2

INGREDIENTS:

- 2 tablespoons olive oil

- 4 skinless, boneless chicken breast cutlets
- ¾ tablespoons black pepper, divided
- ½ teaspoon kosher salt, divided
- 8 oz. mushrooms, sliced
- 4 thyme sprigs
- 0.2 quarts unsalted chicken stock
- quarts Marsala wine
- tablespoons olive oil
- tablespoon fresh thyme, chopped

DIRECTIONS:

1. Heat oil in a pan and fry chicken for 4-5 minutes per side. Remove chicken from the pan and set it aside.
2. In same pan add thyme, mushrooms, salt, and pepper; stir fry for 1-2 minutes.
3. Add Marsala wine, chicken broth, and cooked chicken. Let simmer for 10-12 minutes on low heat.
4. Add to a serving dish.
5. Enjoy.

NUTRITION: Calories – 206, Fat –17 g, Carbs – 3 g, Protein – 8 g

34. Cauliflower Steaks with Eggplant Relish

Preparation Time: 5 minutes

Cooking Time: 25 minutes

Servings: 2

INGREDIENTS:

- 2 small heads cauliflower (about 3 pounds)
- ¼ teaspoon kosher or sea salt
- ¼ teaspoon smoked paprika
- Extra-virgin olive oil, divided

DIRECTIONS:

1. Place a large, rimmed baking sheet in the oven. Preheat the oven to 400°F with the pan inside.

2. Stand one head of cauliflower on a cutting board, stem-end down. With a long chef's knife, slice down through the very center of the head, including the stem.

3. Starting at the cut edge, measure about 1 inch and cut one thick slice from each cauliflower half, including as much of the stem as possible, to make two cauliflower "steaks."

4. Reserve the remaining cauliflower for another use. Repeat with the second cauliflower head.

5. Dry each steak well with a clean towel. Sprinkle the salt and smoked paprika evenly over both sides of each cauliflower steak.

6. In a large skillet over medium-high heat, heat 2 tablespoons of oil. When the oil is very hot, add two cauliflower steaks to the pan and cook for about 3 minutes, until golden and crispy. Flip and cook for 2 more minutes.

7. Transfer the steaks to a plate. Use a pair of tongs to hold a paper towel and wipe out the pan to remove most of the hot oil (which will contain a few burnt bits of cauliflower).

8. Repeat the cooking process with the remaining 2 tablespoons of oil and the remaining two steaks.

9. Using oven mitts, carefully remove the baking sheet from the oven and place the cauliflower on the baking sheet.

10. Roast in the oven for 12 to 15 minutes, until the cauliflower steaks are just fork tender; they will still be somewhat firm. Serve the steaks with the Eggplant Relish Spread, baba ghanoush, or the homemade ketchup.

NUTRITION: Calories – 206, Fat –17 g, Carbs – 3 g, Protein – 8 g

35. Lemon Caper Chicken

Preparation Time: 10 minutes

Cooking Time: 15 minutes

Servings: 2

INGREDIENTS:

- 2 tablespoon virgin olive oil
- 2 chicken breasts (boneless, skinless, cut in half, pound to ¾ an inch thick)
- ¼ cup capers
- 2 lemons (wedges)
- 1 teaspoon oregano
- 1 teaspoon basil
- ½ teaspoon black pepper

DIRECTIONS:

1. Take a large skillet and place it on your stove and add the olive oil to it. Turn the heat to medium and allow it to warm up.

2. As the oil heats up season your chicken breast with the oregano, basil, and black pepper on each side.

3. Place your chicken breast into the hot skillet and cook on each side for five minutes.

4. Transfer the chicken from the skillet to your dinner plate. Top with capers and serve with a few lemon wedges.

NUTRITION: Calories – 182, Carbs - 3.4 g, Protein - 26.6 g, Fat - 8.2 g

36. Herb Roasted Chicken

Preparation Time: 20 minutes

Cooking Time: 45 minutes

Servings: 2

INGREDIENTS:

- 1 tablespoon virgin olive oil
- 1 whole chicken
- 2 rosemary springs
- 3 garlic cloves (peeled)
- 1 lemon (cut in half)
- 1 teaspoon sea salt
- 1 teaspoon black pepper

DIRECTIONS:

1. Turn your oven to 450 degrees F.

2. Take your whole chicken and pat it dry using paper towels. Then rub in the olive oil. Remove the leaves from one of the springs of rosemary and scatter them over the chicken. Sprinkle the sea salt and black pepper over top. Place the other whole sprig of rosemary into the cavity of the chicken. Then add in the garlic cloves and lemon halves.

3. Place the chicken into a roasting pan and then place it into the oven. Allow the chicken to bake for 1 hour, then check that the internal temperature should be at least 165 degrees F. If the chicken begins to brown too much, cover it with foil and return it to the oven to finish cooking.

4. When the chicken has cooked to the appropriate temperature remove it from the oven. Let it rest for at least 20 minutes before carving.

5. Serve with a large side of roasted or steamed vegetables or your favorite salad.

NUTRITION: Calories – 309, Carbs - 1.5 g, Protein - 27.2 g, Fat - 21.3 g

37. Mediterranean bowl

Preparation Time: 25 minutes

Cooking Time: 30 minutes

Servings: 2

INGREDIENTS:

- 2 chicken breasts (chopped into 4 halves)
- 2 diced onions

- 2 bottles of lemon pepper marinade

- 2 diced green bell pepper

- 4 lemon juices

- 8 cloves of crushed garlic.

- 5 teaspoon of olive oil

- Feta cheese

- 1 grape tomato

- 1 large-sized diced zucchini and 1 small-sized. Otherwise, use two medium-sized diced zucchinis.

- Salt and pepper (according to your desired taste), 4 cups of water.

- Kalamata olives (as much as you fancy)

- 1 cup of garbanzo beans

NUTRITION: 541 Cal, 34g of protein, 1423mg of potassium, 12g of fiber, 15g of sugar, 72mg of cholesterol, 4g of fat, 45g of carbs.

38. Tasty Lamb Leg

Preparation Time: 10 minutes

Cooking Time: 20 minutes

Servings: 2

INGREDIENTS:

- 2 lbs. leg of lamb, boneless and cut into chunks

- 1 tbsp. olive oil

- 1 tbsp. garlic, sliced

- 1 cup red wine

- 1 cup onion, chopped

- 2 carrots, chopped

- 1 tsp. rosemary, chopped

- 2 tsp. thyme, chopped

- 1 tsp. oregano, chopped

- 1/2 cup beef stock

- 2 tbsp. tomato paste

- Pepper

- Salt

DIRECTIONS:

1. Add oil into the inner pot of instant pot and set the pot on sauté mode.

2. Add meat and sauté until browned.

3. Add remaining ingredients and stir well.

4. Seal pot with lid and cook on high for 15 minutes.

5. Once done, allow to release pressure naturally. Remove lid.

6. Stir well and serve.

NUTRITION: Calories 540, Fat 20.4 g, Carbohydrates 10.3 g, Sugar 4.2 g, Protein 65.2 g, Cholesterol 204 mg

39. Kale Sprouts & Lamb

Preparation Time: 10 minutes

Cooking Time: 30 minutes

Servings: 2

INGREDIENTS:

- 2 lbs. lamb, cut into chunks
- 1 tbsp. parsley, chopped
- 2 tbsp. olive oil
- 1 cup kale, chopped
- 1 cup Brussels sprouts, halved
- 1 cup beef stock
- Pepper
- Salt

DIRECTIONS:

1. Add all ingredients into the inner pot of instant pot and stir well.
2. Seal pot with lid and cook on high for 30 minutes.
3. Once done, allow to release pressure naturally. Remove lid.
4. Serve and enjoy.

NUTRITION: Calories 504, Fat 23.8 g, Carbohydrates 3.9 g, Sugar 0.5 g, Protein 65.7 g, Cholesterol 204 mg

40. Grilled Harissa Chicken

Preparation Time: 20 minutes

Cooking Time: 12 minutes

Servings: 2

INGREDIENTS:

- Juice of 1 lemon
- 1/2 sliced red onion
- 1 ½ teaspoon of coriander
- 1 ½ teaspoon of smoked paprika

- 1 teaspoon of cumin

- 2 teaspoons of cayenne

- Olive oil

- 1 ½ teaspoon of Black pepper

- Kosher salt

- 5 ounces of thawed and drained frozen spinach

- 8 boneless chickens.

DIRECTIONS:

1. Get a large bowl. Season your chicken with kosher salt on all sides, then add onions, garlic, lemon juice, and harissa paste to the bowl.

2. Add about 3 tablespoons of olive oil to the mixture. Heat a grill to 459 heat (an indoor or outdoor grill works just fine), then oil the grates.

3. Grill each side of the chicken for about 7 minutes. Its temperature should register 165 degrees on a thermometer and it should be fully cooked by then.

NUTRITION: 142.5 kcal, 4.7g of fat, 1.2g of saturated fat, 102mg of sodium, 1.7g of carbs, 107.4mg of cholesterol, 22.1g of protein.

MAIN RECIPES: SEAFOOD

41. Pistachio-Crusted Whitefish

Preparation Time: 10 minutes

Cooking Time: 20 minutes

Servings: 2

INGREDIENTS:

- ¼ cup shelled pistachios
- 1 tablespoon fresh parsley
- 1 tablespoon grated Parmesan cheese
- 1 tablespoon panko bread crumbs
- 2 tablespoons olive oil
- ¼ teaspoon salt
- 10 ounces skinless whitefish (1 large piece or 2 smaller ones)

DIRECTIONS:

1. Preheat the oven to 350°F and set the rack to the middle position. Line a sheet pan with foil or parchment paper.
2. Combine all of the ingredients except the fish in a mini food processor, and pulse until the nuts are finely ground.
3. Alternatively, you can mince the nuts with a chef's knife and combine the ingredients by hand in a small bowl.
4. Place the fish on the sheet pan. Spread the nut mixture evenly over the fish and pat it down lightly.

5. Bake the fish for 20 to 30 minutes, depending on the thickness, until it flakes easily with a fork.

6. Keep in mind that a thicker cut of fish takes a bit longer to bake. You'll know it's done when it's opaque, flakes apart easily with a fork, or reaches an internal temperature of 145°F

NUTRITION: Calories – 185, Carbs - 23.8 g, Protein - 10.1 g, Fat - 5.2 g

42. Crispy Homemade Fish Sticks Recipe

Preparation Time: 10 minutes

Cooking Time: 15 minutes

Servings: 2

INGREDIENTS:

- ½ cup of flour
- 1 beaten egg
- 1 cup of flour
- ½ cup of parmesan cheese
- ½ cup of bread crumbs.
- Zest of 1 lemon juice
- Parsley
- Salt
- 1 teaspoon of black pepper
- 1 tablespoon of sweet paprika
- 1 teaspoon of oregano
- 1 ½ lb. of salmon

- Extra virgin olive oil

DIRECTIONS:

1. Preheat your oven to about 450 degrees F. Get a bowl, dry your salmon and season its two sides with the salt.

2. Then chop into small sizes of 1½ inch length each. Get a bowl and mix black pepper with oregano.

3. Add paprika to the mixture and blend it. Then spice the fish stick with the mixture you have just made. Get another dish and pour your flours.

4. You will need a different bowl again to pour your egg wash into. Pick yet the fourth dish, mix your breadcrumb with your parmesan and add lemon zest to the mixture.

5. Return to the fish sticks and dip each fish into flour such that both sides are coated with flour. As you dip each fish into flour, take it out and dip it into egg wash and lastly, dip it in the breadcrumb mixture.

6. Do this for all fish sticks and arrange on a baking sheet. Ensure you oil the baking sheet before arranging the stick thereon and drizzle the top of the fish sticks with extra virgin olive oil.

7. Caution: allow excess flours to fall off a fish before dipping it into other ingredients.

8. Also ensure that you do not let the coating peel while you add extra virgin olive oil on top of the fishes.

9. Fix the baking sheet in the middle of the oven and allow it to cook for 13 min. By then, the fishes should be golden brown

and you can collect them from the oven, and you can serve immediately.

10. Top it with your lemon zest, parsley and fresh lemon juice.

NUTRITION: 119 Cal, 3.4g of fat, 293.1mg of sodium, 9.3g of carbs, 13.5g of protein.

43. Sauced Shellfish in White Wine

Preparation Time: 10 minutes

Cooking Time: 10 minutes

Servings: 2

INGREDIENTS:

- 2-lbs fresh cuttlefish
- ½-cup olive oil
- 1-pc large onion, finely chopped
- 1-cup of Robola white wine
- ¼-cup lukewarm water
- 1-pc bay leaf
- ½-bunch parsley, chopped
- 4-pcs tomatoes, grated
- Salt and pepper

DIRECTIONS:

1. Take out the hard centerpiece of cartilage (cuttlebone), the bag of ink, and the intestines from the cuttlefish.
2. Wash the cleaned cuttlefish with running water. Slice it into small pieces, and drain excess water.

3. Heat the oil in a saucepan placed over medium-high heat and sauté the onion for 3 minutes until tender.

4. Add the sliced cuttlefish and pour in the white wine. Cook for 5 minutes until it simmers.

5. Pour in the water, and add the tomatoes, bay leaf, parsley, tomatoes, salt, and pepper. Simmer the mixture over low heat until the cuttlefish slices are tender and left with their thick sauce. Serve them warm with rice.

6. Be careful not to overcook the cuttlefish as its texture becomes very hard. A safe rule of thumb is grilling the cuttlefish over a ragingly hot fire for 3 minutes before using it in any recipe.

NUTRITION: Calories: 308, Fats: 18.1g, Dietary Fiber: 1.5g, Carbohydrates: 8g, Protein: 25.6g

44. Pistachio Sole Fish

Preparation Time: 5 minutes

Cooking Time: 10 minutes

Servings: 2

INGREDIENTS:

- 4 (5 ounces) boneless sole fillets
- ½ cup pistachios, finely chopped
- Juice of 1 lemon
- teaspoon extra virgin olive oil

DIRECTIONS:

1. Pre-heat your oven to 350 degrees Fahrenheit

2. Wrap baking sheet using parchment paper and keep it on the side

3. Pat fish dry with kitchen towels and lightly season with salt and pepper

4. Take a small bowl and stir in pistachios

5. Place sol on the prepped sheet and press 2 tablespoons of pistachio mixture on top of each fillet

6. Rub the fish with lemon juice and olive oil

7. Bake for 10 minutes until the top is golden and fish flakes with a fork

NUTRITION: 166 Calories 6g Fat 2g Carbohydrates

45. Speedy Tilapia with Red Onion and Avocado

Preparation time: 10 minutes

Cooking time: 5 minutes

Servings: 2

INGREDIENTS:

- 1 tablespoon extra-virgin olive oil
- 1 tablespoon freshly squeezed orange juice
- ¼ teaspoon kosher or sea salt
- 4 (4-ounces) tilapia fillets, more oblong than square, skin-on or skinned
- ¼ cup chopped red onion (about 1/8 onion)
- 1 avocado, pitted, skinned, and sliced

DIRECTIONS:

1. In a 9-inch glass pie dish, use a fork to mix together the oil, orange juice, and salt. Working with one fillet at a time, place each in the pie dish and turn to coat on all sides.

2. Arrange the fillets in a wagon-wheel formation, so that one end of each fillet is in the center of the dish and the other end is temporarily draped over the edge of the dish.

3. Top each fillet with 1 tablespoon of onion, then fold the end of the fillet that's hanging over the edge in half over the onion.

4. When finished, you should have 4 folded-over fillets with the fold against the outer edge of the dish and the ends all in the center.

5. Cover the dish with plastic wrap, leaving a small part open at the edge to vent the steam. Microwave on high for about 3 minutes.

6. The fish is done when it just begins to separate into flakes (chunks) when pressed gently with a fork. Top the fillets with the avocado and serve.

NUTRITION: 4 g carbohydrates, 3 g fiber, 22 g protein

46. Steamed Mussels in white Wine Sauce

Preparation time: 5 minutes

Cooking time: 10 minutes

Servings: 2

INGREDIENTS:

- 2 pounds small mussels
- 1 tablespoon extra-virgin olive oil

- 1 cup thinly sliced red onion

- 3 garlic cloves, sliced

- 1 cup dry white wine

- 2 (¼-inch-thick) lemon slices

- ¼ teaspoon freshly ground black pepper

- ¼ teaspoon kosher or sea salt

- Fresh lemon wedges, for serving (optional)

DIRECTIONS:

1. In a large colander in the sink, run cold water over the mussels (but don't let the mussels sit in standing water).

2. All the shells should be closed tight; discard any shells that are a little bit open or any shells that are cracked. Leave the mussels in the colander until you're ready to use them.

3. In a large skillet over medium-high heat, heat the oil. Add the onion and cook for 4 minutes, stirring occasionally.

4. Add the garlic and cook for 1 minute, stirring constantly. Add the wine, lemon slices, pepper, and salt, and bring to a simmer. Cook for 2 minutes.

5. Add the mussels and cover. Cook for 3 minutes, or until the mussels open their shells. Gently shake the pan two or three times while they are cooking.

6. All the shells should now be wide open. Using a slotted spoon, discard any mussels that are still closed. Spoon the opened mussels into a shallow serving bowl, and pour the broth over the top. Serve with additional fresh lemon slices, if desired.

NUTRITION: Calories 22, 7 g total fat, 1 g fiber, 18 g protein

47. Orange and Garlic Shrimp

Preparation time: 20 minutes

Cooking time: 10 minutes

Servings: 2

INGREDIENTS:

- 1 large orange
- 3 tablespoons extra-virgin olive oil, divided
- 1 tablespoon chopped fresh Rosemary
- 1 tablespoon chopped fresh thyme
- 3 garlic cloves, minced (about 1½ teaspoons)
- ¼ teaspoon freshly ground black pepper
- ¼ teaspoon kosher or sea salt
- 1½ pounds fresh raw shrimp, shells, and tails removed

DIRECTIONS:

1. Zest the entire orange using a citrus grater. In a large zip-top plastic bag, combine the orange zest and 2 tablespoons of oil with the Rosemary, thyme, garlic, pepper, and salt.

2. Add the shrimp, seal the bag, and gently massage the shrimp until all the ingredients are combined and the shrimp is completely covered with the seasonings. Set aside.

3. Heat a grill, grill pan, or a large skillet over medium heat. Brush on or swirl in the remaining 1 tablespoon of oil.

4. Add half the shrimp, and cook for 4 to 6 minutes, or until the shrimp turn pink and white, flipping halfway through if on the

grill or stirring every minute if in a pan. Transfer the shrimp to a large serving bowl.

5. Repeat with the remaining shrimp, and add them to the bowl.

6. While the shrimp cook, peel the orange and cut the flesh into bite-size pieces. Add to the serving bowl, and toss with the cooked shrimp. Serve immediately or refrigerate and serve cold.

NUTRITION: Calories 190, 8 g total fat, 1 g fiber, 24 g protein

48. Roasted Shrimp-Gnocchi Bake

Preparation time: 10 minutes

Cooking time: 20 minutes

Servings: 2

INGREDIENTS:

- 1 cup chopped fresh tomato
- 2 tablespoons extra-virgin olive oil
- 2 garlic cloves, minced
- ½ teaspoon freshly ground black pepper
- ¼ teaspoon crushed red pepper
- 1 (12-ounces) jar roasted red peppers
- 1-pound fresh raw shrimp, shells and tails removed
- 1-pound frozen gnocchi (not thawed)
- ½ cup cubed feta cheese
- 1/3 cup fresh torn basil leaves

DIRECTIONS:

1. Preheat the oven to 425°F. In a baking dish, mix the tomatoes, oil, garlic, black pepper, and crushed red pepper. Roast in the oven for 10 minutes.

2. Stir in the roasted peppers and shrimp. Roast for 10 more minutes, until the shrimp turn pink and white.

3. While the shrimp cooks, cook the gnocchi on the stovetop according to the package directions.

4. Drain in a colander and keep warm. Remove the dish from the oven. Mix in the cooked gnocchi, feta, and basil, and serve.

NUTRITION: Calories 227, 7 g total fat, 1 g fiber, 20 g protein

49. Spicy Shrimp Puttanesca

Preparation time: 5 minutes

Cooking time: 15 minutes

Servings: 2

INGREDIENTS:

- 2 tablespoons extra-virgin olive oil
- 3 anchovy fillets, drained and chopped
- 3 garlic cloves, minced
- ½ teaspoon crushed red pepper
- 1 (14.5-ounces) can low-sodium or no-salt-added diced tomatoes, undrained
- 1 (2.25-ounces) can sliced black olives, drained
- 2 tablespoons capers
- 1 tablespoon chopped fresh oregano

- 1-pound fresh raw shrimp, shells and tails removed

DIRECTIONS:

1. In a large skillet over medium heat, heat the oil. Mix in the anchovies, garlic, and crushed red pepper.

2. Cook for 3 minutes, stirring frequently and mashing up the anchovies with a wooden spoon until they have melted into the oil.

3. Stir in the tomatoes with their juices, olives, capers, and oregano. Turn up the heat to medium-high, and bring to a simmer.

4. When the sauce is lightly bubbling, stir in the shrimp. Reduce the heat to medium, and cook the shrimp for 6 to 8 minutes, or until they turn pink and white, stirring occasionally, and serve.

NUTRITION: Calories 214, 10 g total fat, 2 g fiber, 26 g protein

50. Baked Cod with Vegetables

Preparation Time: 15 minutes

Cooking Time: 25 minutes

Serving: 2

INGREDIENTS:

- 1 pound (454 g) thick cod fillet, cut into 4 even portions
- ¼ teaspoon onion powder (optional)
- ¼ teaspoon paprika
- 3 tablespoons extra-virgin olive oil
- 4 medium scallions
- ½ cup fresh chopped basil, divided

- 3 tablespoons minced garlic (optional)

- 2 teaspoons salt

- 2 teaspoons freshly ground black pepper

- ¼ teaspoon dry marjoram (optional)

- 6 sun-dried tomato slices

- ½ cup dry white wine

- ½ cup crumbled feta cheese

- 1 (15-ounce / 425-g) can oil-packed artichoke hearts, drained

- 1 lemon, sliced

- 1 cup pitted kalamata olives

- 1 teaspoon capers (optional)

- 4 small red potatoes, quartered

DIRECTION:

1. Set oven to 375°F (190°C).

2. Season the fish with paprika and onion powder (if desired).

3. Heat an ovenproof skillet over medium heat and sear the top side of the cod for about 1 minute until golden. Set aside.

4. Heat the olive oil in the same skillet over medium heat. Add the scallions, ¼ cup of basil, garlic (if desired), salt, pepper, marjoram (if desired), tomato slices, and white wine and stir to combine. Boil then removes from heat.

5. Evenly spread the sauce on the bottom of skillet. Place the cod on top of the tomato basil sauce and scatter with feta cheese. Place the artichokes in the skillet and top with the lemon slices.

6. Scatter with the olives, capers (if desired), and the remaining ¼ cup of basil. Pullout from the heat and transfer to the preheated oven. Bake for 15 to 20 minutes

7. Meanwhile, place the quartered potatoes on a baking sheet or wrapped in aluminum foil. Bake in the oven for 15 minutes.

8. Cool for 5 minutes before serving.

NUTRITION: Calories 1168, 60g fat, 64g protein

51. Slow Cooker Salmon in Foil

Preparation Time: 5 minutes

Cooking Time: 2 hours

Serving: 2

INGREDIENTS:

- 2 (6-ounce / 170-g) salmon fillets
- 1 tablespoon olive oil
- 2 cloves garlic, minced
- ½ tablespoon lime juice
- 1 teaspoon finely chopped fresh parsley
- ¼ teaspoon black pepper

DIRECTION

1. Spread a length of foil onto a work surface and place the salmon fillets in the middle.

2. Blend olive oil, garlic, lime juice, parsley, and black pepper. Brush the mixture over the fillets. Fold the foil over and crimp the sides to make a packet.

3. Place the packet into the slow cooker, cover, and cook on High for 2 hours

4. Serve hot.

NUTRITION: Calories 446, 21g fat, 65g protein

MAIN RECIPES:

VEGETABLE

52. Mediterranean Romaine Wedge Salad

Preparation time: 15 minutes

Cooking time: 0 minutes

Servings: 4

INGREDIENTS:

- 1 English cucumber, chopped
- 1 cup quartered cherry tomatoes
- 1 cup chopped fennel
- ½ cup chopped roasted red peppers
- ¼ cup pitted, halved Kalamata olives
- 1 scallion, both white and green parts, chopped
- ½ cup Pesto Vinaigrette, divided
- 2 romaine lettuce heads, cut in half lengthwise
- ¼ cup grated Asiago cheese
- 2 tablespoons chopped fresh basil

DIRECTIONS:

1. In a large bowl, stir together the cucumber, tomatoes, fennel, roasted red peppers, olives, scallion, and ¼ cup of pesto vinaigrette.

2. Place each romaine half on a large plate. Evenly divide the vegetable mixture onto each wedge. Drizzle the remaining dressing over the romaine wedges. Serve topped with Asiago cheese and basil.

NUTRITION: Calories: 336 Fat: 27g Carbohydrates: 23g Protein: 11g

53. Roasted Brussels Sprouts and Halloumi Salad

Preparation time: 15 minutes

Cooking time: 35 minutes

Servings: 4

INGREDIENTS:

- For the dressing:
- ¼ cup olive oil
- 1/3 cup freshly squeezed lemon juice
- 2 tablespoons honey
- 1 teaspoon mustard
- Sea salt
- Freshly ground black pepper
- For the salad:
- 2 pounds Brussels sprouts, trimmed and halved
- 2 tablespoons olive oil
- 1 teaspoon sea salt
- 1½ cups baby spinach
- ½ cup baby arugula

- 1 shallot, halved and thinly sliced
- 3 tablespoons dried cranberries
- ½ cup blanched almonds, toasted
- ¼ cup shredded halloumi cheese

DIRECTIONS:

1. To Make the Dressing:
2. In a small bowl, whisk together the olive oil, lemon juice, honey, and mustard. Season with salt and pepper and set aside.
3. To Make the Salad:
4. Preheat the oven to 425°F. Put the Brussels sprouts in a large mixing bowl. Drizzle with olive oil and season with salt. Toss to combine.
5. Spread the Brussels sprouts on a large baking sheet. Roast for 25 to 30 minutes, stirring once about halfway through, until crispy on the outside and tender on the inside.
6. While the Brussels sprouts are roasting, in a large mixing bowl, combine the spinach, arugula, shallot, cranberries, and almonds. Once cooked, add the roasted Brussels sprouts to the bowl.
7. Pour the dressing on the salad and toss to combine. Add shredded halloumi cheese and give it another gentle toss. Transfer the salad to a large serving platter.

NUTRITION: Calories: 475 Fat: 34g Carbohydrates: 41g Protein: 14g

54. Roasted Vegetable Mélange

Preparation time: 15 minutes

Cooking time: 25 minutes

Servings: 4

INGREDIENTS:

- ½ cauliflower head, cut into small florets
- ½ broccoli head, cut into small florets
- 2 zucchinis, cut into ½-inch pieces
- 2 cups halved mushrooms
- 2 red, orange, or yellow bell peppers, cut into 1-inch pieces
- 1 sweet potato, cut into 1-inch pieces
- 1 red onion, cut into wedges
- 3 tablespoons olive oil
- 2 teaspoons minced garlic
- 1 teaspoon chopped fresh thyme
- Sea salt
- Freshly ground black pepper

DIRECTIONS:

1. Preheat the oven to 400°F. Line a baking sheet with parchment paper and set aside.
2. In a large bowl, toss the cauliflower, broccoli, zucchini, mushrooms, bell peppers, sweet potato, onion, olive oil, garlic, and thyme until well mixed.
3. Spread the vegetables on the baking sheet and season lightly with salt and pepper. Roast until the vegetables are tender and lightly caramelized, stirring occasionally, 20 to 25 minutes. Serve.

NUTRITION: Calories: 183 Fat: 11g Carbohydrates: 20g Protein: 5g

55. Couscous-Avocado Salad

Preparation time: 15 minutes

Cooking time: 10 minutes

Servings: 4

INGREDIENTS:

- For the dressing:
- ¼ cup olive oil
- 2 tablespoons red wine vinegar
- 1 teaspoon minced garlic
- 1 teaspoon chopped fresh oregano
- Pinch red pepper flakes
- Sea salt
- Freshly ground black pepper
- For the salad:
- 1 cup couscous
- 2 cups halved cherry tomatoes
- ½ English cucumber, chopped
- 1 cup chopped marinated artichoke hearts
- 1 avocado, pitted, peeled, and chopped
- ½ cup crumbled feta cheese
- 2 tablespoons pine nuts

DIRECTIONS:

1. To Make the Dressing:

2. In a small bowl, whisk together the olive oil, vinegar, garlic, oregano, and red pepper flakes. Season with salt and pepper and set aside.

3. To Make the Salad:

4. In a pot, bring 1½ cups of water to a boil. Stir the couscous into the boiling water and remove from the heat. Cover and let sit for 10 minutes. Fluff with a fork.

5. In a large bowl, toss together the couscous, cherry tomatoes, cucumber, artichoke hearts, avocado, feta cheese, and pine nuts. Add the dressing and toss to combine. Refrigerate for 1 hour and serve.

NUTRITION: Calories: 489 Fat: 30g Carbohydrates: 46g Protein: 11g

56. Paprika Cauliflower Steaks with Walnut Sauce

Preparation time: 15 minutes

Cooking time: 30 minutes

Servings: 2

INGREDIENTS:

- Walnut Sauce:
- ½ cup raw walnut halves
- 2 tablespoons virgin olive oil, divided
- 1 clove garlic, chopped
- 1 small yellow onion, chopped
- ½ cup unsweetened almond milk

- 2 tablespoons fresh lemon juice

- Salt and pepper, to taste

- Paprika Cauliflower:

- 1 medium head cauliflower

- 1 teaspoon sweet paprika

- 1 teaspoon minced fresh thyme leaves (about 2 sprigs)

DIRECTIONS:

1. Preheat the oven to 350°F (180°C). Make the walnut sauce: Toast the walnuts in a large, ovenproof skillet over medium heat until fragrant and slightly darkened, about 5 minutes. Transfer the walnuts to a blender.

2. Heat 1 tablespoon of olive oil in the skillet. Add the garlic and onion and sauté for about 2 minutes, or until slightly softened.

3. Transfer the garlic and onion into the blender, along with the almond milk, lemon juice, salt, and pepper. Blend the ingredients until smooth and creamy. Keep the sauce warm while you prepare the cauliflower.

4. Make the paprika cauliflower: Cut two 1-inch-thick "steaks" from the center of the cauliflower. Lightly moisten the steaks with water and season both sides with paprika, thyme, salt, and pepper.

5. Heat the remaining 1 tablespoon of olive oil in the skillet over medium-high heat. Add the cauliflower steaks and sear for about 3 minutes until evenly browned. Flip the cauliflower steaks and transfer the skillet to the oven.

6. Roast in the preheated oven for about 20 minutes until crisp-tender. Serve the cauliflower steaks warm with the walnut sauce on the side.

NUTRITION: Calories: 367 Fat: 27.9g Protein: 7.0g Carbs: 22.7g

57. Stir-Fried Eggplant

Preparation time: 15 minutes

Cooking time: 15 minutes

Servings: 2

INGREDIENTS:

- 1 cup water, plus more as needed
- ½ cup chopped red onion
- 1 tablespoon finely chopped garlic
- 1 tablespoon dried Italian herb seasoning
- 1 teaspoon ground cumin
- 1 small eggplant (about 8 ounces / 227 g), peeled and cut into ½-inch cubes
- 1 medium carrot, sliced
- 2 cups green beans, cut into 1-inch pieces
- 2 ribs celery, sliced
- 1 cup corn kernels
- 2 tablespoons almond butter
- 2 medium tomatoes, chopped

DIRECTIONS:

1. Heat 1 tablespoon of water in a large soup pot over medium-high heat until it sputters. Cook the onion for 2 minutes, adding a little more water as needed.

2. Add the garlic, Italian seasoning, cumin, and eggplant and stir-fry for 2 to 3 minutes, adding a little more water as needed.

3. Add the carrot, green beans, celery, corn kernels, and ½ cup of water and stir well. Reduce the heat to medium, cover, and cook for 8 to 10 minutes, stirring occasionally, or until the vegetables are tender. Meanwhile, in a bowl, stir together the almond butter and ½ cup of water.

4. Remove the vegetables from the heat and stir in the almond butter mixture and chopped tomatoes. Cool for a few minutes before serving.

NUTRITION: Calories: 176 Fat: 5.5g Protein: 5.8g Carbs: 25.4g

58. Simple Honey-Glazed Baby Carrots

Preparation time: 15 minutes

Cooking time: 6 minutes

Servings: 2

INGREDIENTS:

- 2/3 cup water
- 1½ pounds (680 g) baby carrots
- 4 tablespoons almond butter
- ½ cup honey
- 1 teaspoon dried thyme
- 1½ teaspoons dried dill

- Salt, to taste

DIRECTIONS:

1. Pour the water into the Instant Pot and add a steamer basket. Place the baby carrots in the basket. Secure the lid. Select the Manual mode and set the cooking time for 4 minutes at High Pressure.

2. Once cooking is complete, do a quick pressure release. Carefully open the lid. Transfer the carrots to a plate and set aside. Pour the water out of the Instant Pot and dry it.

3. Press the Sauté button on the Instant Pot and heat the almond butter. Stir in the honey, thyme, and dill.

4. Return the carrots to the Instant Pot and stir until well coated. Sauté for another 1 minute. Taste and season with salt as needed. Serve warm.

NUTRITION: Calories: 575 Fat: 23.5g Protein: 2.8g Carbs: 90.6g

59. Quick Steamed Broccoli

Preparation time: 15 minutes

Cooking time: 0 minutes

Servings: 2

INGREDIENTS:

- ¼ cup water
- 3 cups broccoli florets
- Salt and ground black pepper, to taste

DIRECTIONS:

1. Pour the water into the Instant Pot and insert a steamer basket. Place the broccoli florets in the basket.

2. Secure the lid. Select the Manual mode and set the cooking time for 0 minutes at High Pressure. Once cooking is complete, do a quick pressure release. Carefully open the lid.

3. Transfer the broccoli florets to a bowl with cold water to keep bright green color. Season the broccoli with salt and pepper to taste, then serve.

NUTRITION: Calories: 16 Fat: 0.2g Protein: 1.9g Carbs: 1.7g

60. Garlic-Butter Asparagus with Parmesan

Preparation time: 5 minutes

Cooking time: 8 minutes

Servings: 2

INGREDIENTS:

- 1 cup water
- 1 pound (454 g) asparagus, trimmed
- 2 cloves garlic, chopped
- 3 tablespoons almond butter
- Salt and ground black pepper, to taste
- 3 tablespoons grated Parmesan cheese

DIRECTIONS:

1. Pour the water into the Instant Pot and insert a trivet. Put the asparagus on a tin foil add the butter and garlic. Season to taste with salt and pepper.

2. Fold over the foil and seal the asparagus inside so the foil doesn't come open. Arrange the asparagus on the trivet.

3. Secure the lid. Select the Manual mode and set the cooking time for 8 minutes at High Pressure. Once cooking is complete, do a quick pressure release. Carefully open the lid.

4. Unwrap the foil packet and serve sprinkled with the Parmesan cheese.

NUTRITION: Calories: 243 Fat: 15.7g Protein: 12.3g Carbs: 15.3g

61. Cucumber Watermelon Salad

Preparation time: 10 minutes

Cooking time: 10 minutes

Servings: 6

INGREDIENTS:

- For salad:
- ½ cup feta cheese, crumbled
- ¼ cup fresh basil leaves, chopped
- ¼ cup fresh mint leaves, chopped
- 1 cucumber, cubed
- ½ watermelon, peeled and cut into cubes
- For dressing:
- 1 tbsp olive oil

- 2 tbsp fresh lime juice
- 2 tbsp honey
- Pinch of salt

DIRECTIONS:

1. In a small bowl, mix together all dressing ingredients and set aside. Add all salad ingredients into the mixing bowl and mix well.

2. Pour dressing over salad and toss well. Serve and enjoy.

NUTRITION: Calories: 130 Fat: 7.6g Protein: 3.5g Carbs: 13.9g

PIZZA RECIPES

62. Basil & Artichoke Pizza

Preparation time: 1 hours & 15 minutes

Cooking time: 24 minutes

Servings: 4

INGREDIENTS:

- 1 cup canned passata
- 2 cups flour
- 1 cup lukewarm water
- 1 pinch of sugar
- 1 tsp active dry yeast
- ¾ tsp salt
- 2 tbsp olive oil
- 1 ½ cups frozen artichoke hearts
- ¼ cup grated Asiago cheese
- ½ onion, minced
- 3 garlic cloves, minced
- 1 tbsp dried oregano
- 1 cup sun-dried tomatoes, chopped
- ½ tsp red pepper flakes
- 5-6 basil leaves, torn

DIRECTIONS:

1. Sift the flour and salt in a bowl and stir in yeast. Mix lukewarm water, olive oil, and sugar in another bowl. Add the wet mixture to the dry mixture and whisk until you obtain a soft dough.

2. Place the dough on a lightly floured work surface and knead it thoroughly for 4-5 minutes until elastic. Transfer the dough to a greased bowl.

3. Cover with cling film and leave to rise for 50-60 minutes in a warm place until doubled in size. Roll out the dough to a thickness of around 12 inches.

4. Preheat oven to 400 F. Warm oil in a saucepan over medium heat and sauté onion and garlic for 3-4 minutes. Mix in tomatoes and oregano and bring to a boil.

5. Decrease the heat and simmer for another 5 minutes. Transfer the pizza crust to a baking sheet. Spread the sauce all over and top with artichoke hearts and sun-dried tomatoes.

6. Scatter the cheese and bake for 15 minutes until golden. Top with red pepper flakes and basil leaves and serve sliced.

NUTRITION: Calories 254 Fat 9.5g Carbs 34.3g Protein 8g

63. Balsamic-Glazed Pizza with Arugula & Olives

Preparation time: 1 hour & 20 minutes

Cooking time: 20 minutes

Servings: 4

INGREDIENTS:

- 2 cups flour

- 1 cup lukewarm water
- 1 pinch of sugar
- 1 tsp active dry yeast
- 2 tbsp olive oil
- 2 tbsp honey
- ½ cup balsamic vinegar
- 4 cups arugula
- Salt and black pepper to taste
- 1 cup mozzarella cheese, grated
- ¾ tsp dried oregano
- 6 black olives, drained

DIRECTIONS:

1. Sift the flour and ¾ tsp salt in a bowl and stir in yeast. Mix lukewarm water, olive oil, and sugar in another bowl. Add the wet mixture to the dry mixture and whisk until you obtain a soft dough.

2. Place the dough on a lightly floured work surface and knead it thoroughly for 4-5 minutes until elastic. Transfer the dough to a greased bowl.

3. Cover with cling film and leave to rise for 50-60 minutes in a warm place until doubled in size. Roll out the dough to a thickness of around 12 inches.

4. Place the balsamic vinegar and honey in a saucepan over medium heat and simmer for 5 minutes until syrupy. Preheat oven to 390 F.

5. Transfer the pizza crust to a baking sheet and sprinkle with oregano and mozzarella cheese; bake for 10-15 minutes.

6. Remove the pizza from the oven and top with arugula. Sprinkle with balsamic glaze and black olives and serve.

NUTRITION: Calories 350 Fat 15.4g Carbs 47.1g Protein 6.4g

64. Pepperoni Fat Head Pizza

Preparation time: 1 hour & 20 minutes

Cooking time: 15 minutes

Servings: 4

INGREDIENTS:

- 2 cups flour
- 1 cup lukewarm water
- 1 pinch of sugar
- 1 tsp active dry yeast
- ¾ tsp salt
- 2 tbsp olive oil
- 1 tsp dried oregano
- 2 cups mozzarella cheese
- 1 cup sliced pepperoni

DIRECTIONS:

1. Sift the flour and salt in a bowl and stir in yeast. Mix lukewarm water, olive oil, and sugar in another bowl. Add the wet mixture to the dry mixture and whisk until you obtain a soft dough.

2. Place the dough on a lightly floured work surface and knead it thoroughly for 4-5 minutes until elastic. Transfer the dough to a greased bowl.

3. Cover with cling film and leave to rise for 50-60 minutes in a warm place until doubled in size. Roll out the dough to a thickness of around 12 inches.

4. Preheat oven to 400 F. Line a round pizza pan with parchment paper. Spread the dough on the pizza pan and top with the mozzarella cheese, oregano, and pepperoni slices.

5. Bake in the oven for 15 minutes or until the cheese melts. Remove the pizza, slice and serve.

NUTRITION: Calories 229 Fats 7.1g Carbs 0.4g Protein 36.4g

65. Extra Cheesy Pizza

Preparation time: 15 minutes

Cooking time: 28 minutes

Servings: 4

INGREDIENTS:

- For the crust:
- ½ cup almond flour
- ¼ tsp salt
- 2 tbsp ground psyllium husk
- 1 tbsp olive oil
- 1 cup lukewarm water
- For the topping

- ½ cup sugar-free pizza sauce
- 1 cup sliced mozzarella cheese
- 1 cup grated mozzarella cheese
- 3 tbsp grated Parmesan cheese
- 2 tsp Italian seasoning

DIRECTIONS:

1. Preheat the oven to 400 F. Line a baking sheet with parchment paper. In a medium bowl, mix the almond flour, salt, psyllium powder, olive oil, and lukewarm water until dough forms.

2. Spread the mixture on the pizza pan and bake in the oven until crusty, 10 minutes. When ready, remove the crust and spread the pizza sauce on top.

3. Add the sliced mozzarella, grated mozzarella, Parmesan cheese, and Italian seasoning. Bake in the oven for 18 minutes or until the cheeses melt. Serve warm.

NUTRITION: Calories 193 Fats 10.2g Carbs 3.2g Protein 19.5g

66. Spanish-Style Pizza de Jamon

Preparation time: 1 hour & 15 minutes

Cooking time: 15 minutes

Servings: 4

INGREDIENTS:

- For the crust:
- 2 cups flour
- 1 cup lukewarm water

- 1 pinch of sugar
- 1 tsp active dry yeast
- ¾ tsp salt
- 2 tbsp olive oil
- For the topping:
- ½ cup tomato sauce
- ½ cup sliced mozzarella cheese
- 4 oz jamon serrano, sliced
- 7 fresh basil leaves

DIRECTIONS:

1. Sift the flour and salt in a bowl and stir in yeast. Mix lukewarm water, olive oil, and sugar in another bowl. Add the wet mixture to the dry mixture and whisk until you obtain a soft dough.

2. Place the dough on a lightly floured work surface and knead it thoroughly for 4-5 minutes until elastic. Transfer the dough to a greased bowl.

3. Cover with cling film and leave to rise for 50-60 minutes in a warm place until doubled in size. Roll out the dough to a thickness of around 12 inches.

4. Preheat the oven to 400 F. Line a pizza pan with parchment paper. Spread the tomato sauce on the crust.

5. Arrange the mozzarella slices on the sauce and then the jamon serrano. Bake for 15 minutes or until the cheese melts. Remove from the oven and top with the basil. Slice and serve warm.

NUTRITION: Calories 160 Fats 6.2g Carbs 0.5g Protein 21.9g

67. Spicy & Smoky Pizza

Preparation time: 1 hour & 15 minutes

Cooking time: 20 minutes

Servings: 4

INGREDIENTS:

- For the crust:
- 2 cups flour
- 1 cup lukewarm water
- 1 pinch of sugar
- 1 tsp active dry yeast
- ¾ tsp salt
- 2 tbsp olive oil
- For the topping:
- 1 tbsp olive oil
- 1 cup sliced chorizo
- ¼ cup sugar-free marinara sauce
- 1 cup sliced smoked mozzarella cheese
- 1 jalapeño pepper, deseeded and sliced
- ¼ red onion, thinly sliced

DIRECTIONS:

1. Sift the flour and salt in a bowl and stir in yeast. Mix lukewarm water, olive oil, and sugar in another bowl. Add the wet mixture to the dry mixture and whisk until you obtain a soft dough.

2. Place the dough on a lightly floured work surface and knead it thoroughly for 4-5 minutes until elastic. Transfer the dough to a greased bowl.

3. Cover with cling film and leave to rise for 50-60 minutes in a warm place until doubled in size. Roll out the dough to a thickness of around 12 inches.

4. Preheat the oven to 400 F. Line a pizza pan with parchment paper. Heat the olive oil and cook the chorizo until brown, 5 minutes.

5. Spread the marinara sauce on the crust, top with the mozzarella cheese, chorizo, jalapeño pepper, and onion.

6. Bake in the oven until the cheese melts, 15 minutes. Remove from the oven, slice, and serve warm.

NUTRITION: Calories 302 Fats 17g Carbs 1.4g Protein 31.6g

68. Turkey Pizza with Pesto Topping

Preparation time: 15 minutes

Cooking time: 30 minutes

Servings: 4

INGREDIENTS:

- Pizza Crust:
- 3 cups flour
- 3 tbsp olive oil
- 1/3 tsp salt
- 3 large eggs
- Pesto Chicken Topping:

- ½ lb. turkey ham, chopped

- 2 tbsp cashew nuts

- Salt and black pepper to taste

- 1 ½ tbsp olive oil

- 1 green bell pepper, seeded and sliced

- 1 ½ cups basil pesto

- 1 cup mozzarella cheese, grated

- 1 ½ tbsp Parmesan cheese, grated

- 1½ tbsp fresh basil leaves

- A pinch of red pepper flakes

DIRECTIONS:

1. In a bowl, mix flour, 3 tbsp of olive oil, salt, and eggs until a dough form. Mold the dough into a ball and place it in between two full parchment papers on a flat surface.

2. Roll it out into a circle of a ¼ -inch thickness. After, slide the pizza dough into the pizza pan and remove the parchment paper. Place the pizza pan in the oven and bake the dough for 20 minutes at 350°F.

3. Once the pizza bread is ready, remove it from the oven, fold and seal the extra inch of dough at its edges to make a crust around it.

4. Apply 2/3 of the pesto on it and sprinkle half of the mozzarella cheese too. Toss the chopped turkey ham in the remaining pesto and spread it on top of the pizza.

5. Sprinkle with the remaining mozzarella, bell peppers, and cashew nuts and put the pizza back in the oven to bake for 9 minutes.

6. When it is ready, remove from the oven to cool slightly, garnish with the basil leaves and sprinkle with parmesan cheese and red pepper flakes. Slice and serve.

NUTRITION: Calories 684 Fat 54g Carbs 22g Protein 31.5g

69. Baby Spinach Pizza with Sweet Onion

Preparation time: 1 hour & 15 minutes

Cooking time: 53 minutes

Servings: 4

INGREDIENTS:

- For the crust:
- 2 cups flour
- 1 cup lukewarm water
- 1 pinch of sugar
- 1 tsp active dry yeast
- ¾ tsp salt
- 2 tbsp olive oil
- For the caramelized onion:
- 1 onion, sliced
- 1 tsp sugar
- 2 tbsp olive oil
- ½ tsp salt

- For the pizza:
- ¼ cup shaved Pecorino Romano cheese
- 2 tbsp olive oil
- ½ cup grated mozzarella cheese
- 1 cup baby spinach
- ¼ cup chopped fresh basil leaves
- ½ red bell pepper, sliced

DIRECTIONS:

1. Sift the flour and salt in a bowl and stir in yeast. Mix lukewarm water, olive oil, and sugar in another bowl. Add the wet mixture to the dry mixture and whisk until you obtain a soft dough.

2. Place the dough on a lightly floured work surface and knead it thoroughly for 4-5 minutes until elastic. Transfer the dough to a greased bowl.

3. Cover with cling film and leave to rise for 50-60 minutes in a warm place until doubled in size. Roll out the dough to a thickness of around 12 inches.

4. Warm olive oil in a skillet over medium heat and sauté onion with salt and sugar for 3 minutes. Lower the heat and brown for 20-35 minutes until caramelized. Preheat oven to 390 F.

5. Transfer the pizza crust to a baking sheet. Drizzle the crust with olive oil and top with onion. Cover with bell pepper and mozzarella. Bake for 10-15 minutes. Serve topped with baby spinach, basil, and Pecorino cheese.

NUTRITION: Calories 399 Fat 22.7g Carbs 42.9g Protein 8.1g

70. Italian Mushroom Pizza

Preparation time: 1 hour & 15 minutes

Cooking time: 25 minutes

Servings: 4

INGREDIENTS:

- For the crust:
- 2 cups flour
- 1 cup lukewarm water
- 1 pinch of sugar
- 1 tsp active dry yeast
- ¾ tsp salt
- 2 tbsp olive oil
- For the topping:
- 1 tsp olive oil
- 2 medium cremini mushrooms, sliced
- 1 garlic clove, minced
- ½ cup sugar-free tomato sauce
- 1 tsp sugar
- 1 bay leaf
- 1 tsp dried oregano
- 1tsp dried basil
- Salt and black pepper to taste
- ½ cup grated mozzarella cheese
- ½ cup grated Parmesan cheese

- 6 black olives, pitted and sliced

DIRECTIONS:

1. Sift the flour and salt in a bowl and stir in yeast. Mix lukewarm water, olive oil, and sugar in another bowl. Add the wet mixture to the dry mixture and whisk until you obtain a soft dough.

2. Place the dough on a lightly floured work surface and knead it thoroughly for 4-5 minutes until elastic. Transfer the dough to a greased bowl.

3. Cover with cling film and leave to rise for 50-60 minutes in a warm place until doubled in size. Roll out the dough to a thickness of around 12 inches.

4. Preheat the oven to 400 F. Line a pizza pan with parchment paper. Heat the olive oil in a medium skillet and sauté the mushrooms until softened, 5 minutes. Stir in the garlic and cook until fragrant, 30 seconds.

5. Mix in the tomato sauce, sugar, bay leaf, oregano, basil, salt, and black pepper. Cook for 2 minutes and turn the heat off.

6. Spread the sauce on the crust, top with the mozzarella and Parmesan cheeses, and then, the olives. Bake in the oven until the cheese's melts, 15 minutes. Remove the pizza, slice, and serve warm.

NUTRITION: Calories 203 Fats 8.6g Carbs 2.6g Protein 24.3g

71. Broccoli-Pepper Pizza

Preparation time: 15 minutes

Cooking time: 20 minutes

Servings: 4

INGREDIENTS:

- For the crust:
- ½ cup almond flour
- ¼ tsp salt
- 2 tbsp ground psyllium husk
- 1 tbsp olive oil
- 1 cup lukewarm water
- For the topping:
- 1 tbsp olive oil
- 1 cup sliced fresh mushrooms
- 1 white onion, thinly sliced
- 3 cups broccoli florets
- 4 garlic cloves, minced
- ½ cup pizza sauce
- 4 tomatoes, sliced
- 1 ½ cup grated mozzarella cheese
- ½ cup grated Parmesan cheese

DIRECTIONS:

1. Preheat the oven to 400 F. Line a baking sheet with parchment paper. In a bowl, mix the almond flour, salt, psyllium powder, olive oil, and lukewarm water until dough forms.

2. Spread the mixture on the pizza pan and bake in the oven until crusty, 10 minutes. When ready, remove the crust and allow cooling.

3. Heat olive oil in a skillet and sauté the mushrooms, onion, garlic, and broccoli until softened, 5 minutes.

4. Spread the pizza sauce on the crust and top with the broccoli mixture, tomato, mozzarella and Parmesan cheeses. Bake for 5 minutes.

NUTRITION: Calories 180 Fats 9g Carbs 3.6g Protein 17g

PASTA RECIPES

72. Pesto Pasta and Shrimps

Preparation time: 15 minutes

Cooking time: 0 minutes

Servings: 4

INGREDIENTS:

- ¼ cup pesto, divided
- ¼ cup shaved Parmesan Cheese
- 1 ¼ lbs. large shrimp, peeled and deveined
- 1 cup halved grape tomatoes
- 4-oz angel hair pasta, cooked, rinsed and drained

DIRECTIONS:

1. On medium high fire, place a nonstick large fry pan and grease with cooking spray. Add tomatoes, pesto and shrimp. Cook for 15 minutes or until shrimps are opaque, while covered.

2. Stir in cooked pasta and cook until heated through. Transfer to a serving plate and garnish with Parmesan cheese.

NUTRITION: Calories: 319 Carbs: 23.6g Protein: 31.4g Fat: 11g

73. Prosciutto E Faggioli

Preparation time: 15 minutes

Cooking time: 5 minutes

Servings: 4

INGREDIENTS:

- 12 oz pasta, cooked and drained
- Pepper and salt to taste
- 3 tbsp snipped fresh chives
- 3 cups arugula or watercress leaves, loosely packed
- ½ cup chicken broth, warm
- 1 tbsp Herbed garlic butter
- ½ cup shredded pecorino Toscano
- 4 oz prosciutto, cut into bite sizes
- 2 cups cherry tomatoes, halved
- 1 can of 19oz white kidney beans, rinsed and drained

DIRECTIONS:

1. Heat over medium low fire herbed garlic butter, cheese, prosciutto, tomatoes and beans in a big saucepan for 2 minutes.
2. Once mixture is simmering, stir constantly to melt cheese while gradually stirring in the broth.
3. Once cheese is fully melted and incorporated, add chives, arugula, pepper and salt. Turn off the fire and toss in the cooked pasta. Serve and enjoy.

NUTRITION: Calories: 452 Carbs: 57.9g Protein: 30.64g Fat: 11.7g

74. Puttanesca Style Bucatini

Preparation time: 15 minutes

Cooking time: 20 minutes

Servings: 4

INGREDIENTS:

- 1 tbsp capers, rinsed
- 1 tsp coarsely chopped fresh oregano
- 1 tsp finely chopped garlic
- 1/8 tsp salt
- 12-oz bucatini pasta
- 2 cups coarsely chopped canned no-salt-added whole peeled tomatoes with their juice
- 3 tbsp extra virgin olive oil, divided
- 4 anchovy fillets, chopped
- 8 black Kalamata olives, pitted and sliced into slivers

DIRECTIONS:

1. Cook bucatini pasta according to package directions. Drain, keep warm, and set aside. On medium fire, place a large nonstick saucepan and heat 2 tbsp oil.
2. Sauté anchovies until it starts to disintegrate. Add garlic and sauté for 15 seconds. Add tomatoes, sauté for 15 to 20 minutes or until no longer watery. Season with 1/8 tsp salt.
3. Add oregano, capers, and olives. Add pasta, sautéing until heated through. To serve, drizzle pasta with remaining olive oil and enjoy.

NUTRITION: Calories: 207.4 Carbs: 31g Protein: 5.1g Fat: 7g

75. Raw Tomato Sauce & Brie on Linguine

Preparation time: 15 minutes

Cooking time: 20 minutes

Servings: 4

INGREDIENTS:

- ¼ cup grated low-fat Parmesan cheese
- ½ cup loosely packed fresh basil leaves, torn
- 12 oz whole wheat linguine
- 2 cups loosely packed baby arugula
- 2 green onions, green parts only, sliced thinly
- 2 tbsp balsamic vinegar
- 2 tbsp extra virgin olive oil
- 3 large vine-ripened tomatoes
- 3 oz low-fat Brie cheese, cubed, rind removed and discarded
- 3 tbsp toasted pine nuts
- Pepper and salt to taste

DIRECTIONS:

1. Toss together pepper, salt, vinegar, oil, onions, Parmesan, basil, arugula, Brie and tomatoes in a large bowl and set aside. Cook linguine following package instructions.

2. Reserve 1 cup of pasta cooking water after linguine is cooked. Drain and discard the rest of the pasta. Do not run under cold water, instead immediately add into bowl of salad.

3. Let it stand for a minute without mixing. Add ¼ cup of reserved pasta water into bowl to make a creamy sauce. Add more pasta water if desired. Toss to mix well. Serve and enjoy.

NUTRITION: Calories: 274.7 Carbs: 30.9g Protein: 14.6g Fat: 10.3g

76. Ricotta and Spinach Ravioli

Preparation time: 15 minutes

Cooking time: 15 minutes

Servings: 2

INGREDIENTS:

- 1 cup chicken stock
- 1 cup frozen spinach, thawed
- 1 batch pasta dough
- Filling:
- 3 tbsp heavy cream
- 1 cup ricotta
- 1 ¾ cups baby spinach
- 1 small onion, finely chopped
- 2 tbsp butter

DIRECTIONS:

1. Create the filling:
2. In a fry pan, sauté onion and butter around five minutes. Add the baby spinach leaves and continue simmering for another four minutes.

3. Remove from fire, drain liquid and mince the onion and leaves. Then combine with 2 tbsp cream and the ricotta ensuring that it is well combined. Add pepper and salt to taste.

4. With your pasta dough, divide it into four balls. Roll out one ball to ¼ inch thick rectangular spread. Cut a 1 ½ inch by 3-inch rectangles.

5. Place filling on the middle of the rectangles, around 1 tablespoonful and brush filling with cold water.

6. Fold the rectangles in half, ensuring that no air is trapped within and seal using a cookie cutter. Use up all the filling.

7. Create Pasta Sauce:

8. Until smooth, puree chicken stock and spinach. Pour into heated fry pan and for two minutes cook it. Add 1 tbsp cream and season with pepper and salt.

9. Continue cooking for a minute and turn of fire. Cook the raviolis by submerging in a boiling pot of water with salt.

10. Cook until al dente then drains. Then quickly transfer the cooked ravioli into the fry pan of pasta sauce, toss to mix and serve.

NUTRITION: Calories: 443 Carbs: 12.3g Protein: 18.8g Fat: 36.8g

77. Roasted Red Peppers and Shrimp Pasta

Preparation time: 15 minutes

Cooking time: 10 minutes

Servings: 6

INGREDIENTS:

- 12 oz pasta, cooked and drained
- 1 cup finely shredded Parmesan Cheese
- ¼ cup snipped fresh basil
- ½ cup whipping cream
- ½ cup dry white wine
- 1 12oz jar roasted red sweet peppers, drained and chopped
- ¼ tsp crushed red pepper
- 6 cloves garlic, minced
- 1/3 cup finely chopped onion
- 2 tbsp olive oil
- ¼ cup butter
- 1 ½ lbs. fresh, peeled, deveined, rinsed and drained medium shrimps

DIRECTIONS:

1. On medium high fire, heat butter in a big fry pan and add garlic and onions. Stir fry until onions are soft, around two minutes.

2. Add crushed red pepper and shrimps, sauté for another two minutes before adding wine and roasted peppers.

3. Allow mixture to boil before lowering heat to low fire and for two minutes, let the mixture simmer uncovered. Stirring occasionally, add cream once shrimps are cooked and simmer for a minute.

4. Add basil and remove from fire. Toss in the pasta and mix gently. Transfer to serving plates and top with cheese.

NUTRITION: Calories: 418 Carbs: 26.9g Protein: 37.1g Fat: 18.8g

78. Seafood and Veggie Pasta

Preparation time: 15 minutes

Cooking time: 10 minutes

Servings: 4

INGREDIENTS:

- ¼ tsp pepper
- ¼ tsp salt
- 1 lb. raw shelled shrimp
- 1 lemon, cut into wedges
- 1 tbsp butter
- 1 tbsp olive oil
- 2 5-oz cans chopped clams, drained (reserve 2 tbsp clam juice)
- 2 tbsp dry white wine
- 4 cloves garlic, minced
- 4 cups zucchini, spiraled (use a veggie spiralizer)
- 4 tbsp Parmesan Cheese
- fresh parsley, chopped to garnish

DIRECTIONS:

1. Ready the zucchini and spiralize with a veggie spiralizer. Arrange 1 cup of zucchini noodle per bowl. Total of 4 bowls.

2. On medium fire, place a large nonstick saucepan and heat oil and butter. For a minute, sauté garlic. Add shrimp and cook for 3 minutes until opaque or cooked.

3. Add white wine, reserved clam juice and clams. Bring to a simmer and continue simmering for 2 minutes or until half of liquid has evaporated. Stir constantly.

4. Season with pepper and salt. Remove from fire and evenly distribute seafood sauce to 4 bowls. Top with a tablespoonful of Parmesan cheese per bowl, serve and enjoy.

NUTRITION: Calories: 324.9 Carbs: 12g Protein: 43.8g Fat: 11.3g

79. Seafood Paella with Couscous

Preparation time: 15 minutes

Cooking time: 10 minutes

Servings: 4

INGREDIENTS:

- ½ cup whole wheat couscous
- 4 oz small shrimp, peeled and deveined
- 4 oz bay scallops, tough muscle removed
- ¼ cup vegetable broth
- 1 cup freshly diced tomatoes and juice
- Pinch of crumbled saffron threads
- ¼ tsp freshly ground pepper
- ¼ tsp salt
- ½ tsp fennel seed
- ½ tsp dried thyme
- 1 clove garlic, minced
- 1 medium onion, chopped

- 2 tsp extra virgin olive oil

DIRECTIONS:

1. Put on medium fire a large saucepan and add oil. Stir in the onion and sauté for three minutes before adding: saffron, pepper, salt, fennel seed, thyme, and garlic.

2. Continue to sauté for another minute. Then add the broth and tomatoes and let boil. Once boiling, reduce the fire, cover and continue to cook for another 2 minutes.

3. Add the scallops and increase fire to medium and stir occasionally and cook for two minutes. Add the shrimp and wait for two minutes more before adding the couscous.

4. Then remove from fire, cover and set aside for five minutes before carefully mixing.

NUTRITION: Calories: 117 Carbs: 11.7g Protein: 11.5g Fat: 3.1g

80. Shrimp Paella Made with Quinoa

Preparation time: 15 minutes

Cooking time: 25 minutes

Servings: 7

INGREDIENTS:

- 1 lb. large shrimp, peeled, deveined and thawed
- 1 tsp seafood seasoning
- 1 cup frozen green peas
- 1 red bell pepper, cored, seeded & membrane removed, sliced into ½" strips
- ½ cup sliced sun-dried tomatoes, packed in olive oil

- Salt to taste

- ½ tsp black pepper

- ½ tsp Spanish paprika

- ½ tsp saffron threads (optional turmeric)

- 1 bay leaf

- ¼ tsp crushed red pepper flakes

- 3 cups chicken broth, fat free, low sodium

- 1 ½ cups dry quinoa, rinse well

- 1 tbsp olive oil

- 2 cloves garlic, minced

- 1 yellow onion, diced

DIRECTIONS:

1. Season shrimps with seafood seasoning and a pinch of salt. Toss to mix well and refrigerate until ready to use. Prepare and wash quinoa. Set aside.

2. On medium low fire, place a large nonstick skillet and heat oil. Add onions and for 5 minutes sauté until soft and tender.

3. Add paprika, saffron (or turmeric), bay leaves, red pepper flakes, chicken broth and quinoa. Season with salt and pepper. Cover skillet and bring to a boil.

4. Once boiling, lower fire to a simmer and cook until all liquid is absorbed, around ten minutes. Add shrimp, peas and sun-dried tomatoes.

5. For 5 minutes, cover and cook. Once done, turn off fire and for ten minutes allow paella to set while still covered. To serve, remove bay leaf and enjoy with a squeeze of lemon if desired.

NUTRITION: Calories: 324.4 Protein: 22g Carbs: 33g Fat: 11.6g

81. Shrimp, Lemon and Basil Pasta

Preparation time: 15 minutes

Cooking time: 0 minutes

Servings: 4

INGREDIENTS:

- 2 cups baby spinach
- ½ tsp salt
- 2 tbsp fresh lemon juice
- 2 tbsp extra virgin olive oil
- 3 tbsp drained capers
- ¼ cup chopped fresh basil
- 1 lb. peeled and deveined large shrimp
- 8 oz uncooked spaghetti
- 3 quarts water

DIRECTIONS:

1. In a pot, bring to boil 3 quarts water. Add the pasta and allow to boil for another eight mins before adding the shrimp and boiling for another three mins or until pasta is cooked.

2. Drain the pasta and transfer to a bowl. Add salt, lemon juice, olive oil, capers and basil while mixing well. To serve, place baby spinach on plate around ½ cup and topped with ½ cup of pasta.

NUTRITION: Calories: 151 Carbs: 18.9g Protein: 4.3g Fat: 7.4g

SNACK RECIPES

82. Greek Salad Wraps

Preparation Time: 15 minutes

Cooking Time: 10 minutes

Servings: 2

INGREDIENTS:

- 1½ cups seedless cucumber, peeled and chopped (about 1 large cucumber)
- 1 cup chopped tomato (about 1 large tomato)
- ½ cup finely chopped fresh mint
- 1 (2.25-ounce) can sliced black olives (about ½ cup), drained
- ¼ cup diced red onion (about ¼ onion)
- 2 tablespoons extra-virgin olive oil
- 1 tablespoon red wine vinegar
- ¼ teaspoon freshly ground black pepper
- ¼ teaspoon kosher or sea salt
- ½ cup crumbled goat cheese (about 2 ounces)
- 4 whole-wheat flatbread wraps or soft whole-wheat tortillas

DIRECTIONS:

1. In a large bowl, mix together the cucumber, tomato, mint, olives, and onion until well combined.

2. In a small bowl, whisk together the oil, vinegar, pepper, and salt. Drizzle the dressing over the salad, and mix gently.

3. With a knife, spread the goat cheese evenly over the four wraps. Spoon a quarter of the salad filling down the middle of each wrap.

4. Fold up each wrap: Start by folding up the bottom, then fold one side over and fold the other side over the top. Repeat with the remaining wraps and serve.

NUTRITION: Calories: 262; Total Fat: 15g; Saturated Fat: 5g; Cholesterol: 15mg; Sodium: 529mg; Total Carbohydrates: 23g; Fiber: 4g; Protein: 7g

83. Dill Salmon Salad Wraps

Preparation Time: 20 minutes

Cooking Time: 60 minutes

Servings: 2

INGREDIENTS:

- 1-pound salmon filet, cooked and flaked, or 3 (5-ounce) cans salmon
- ½ cup diced carrots (about 1 carrot)
- ½ cup diced celery (about 1 celery stalk)
- 3 tablespoons chopped fresh dill
- 3 tablespoons diced red onion (a little less than 1/8 onion)
- 2 tablespoons capers
- 1½ tablespoons extra-virgin olive oil

- 1 tablespoon aged balsamic vinegar
- ½ teaspoon freshly ground black pepper
- ¼ teaspoon kosher or sea salt
- 4 whole-wheat flatbread wraps or soft whole-wheat tortillas

DIRECTIONS:

1. In a large bowl, mix together the salmon, carrots, celery, dill, red onion, capers, oil, vinegar, pepper, and salt.
2. Divide the salmon salad among the flatbreads. Fold up the bottom of the flatbread, then roll up the wrap and serve.

NUTRITION: Calories: 336; Total Fat: 16g; Saturated Fat: 2g; Cholesterol: 67mg; Sodium: 628mg; Total Carbohydrates: 23g; Fiber: 5g; Protein: 32g

84. Chicken Parmesan Wraps

Preparation Time: 10 minutes

Cooking Time: 20 minutes

Servings: 2

INGREDIENTS:

- Nonstick cooking spray
- 1-pound boneless, skinless chicken breasts
- 1 large egg
- ¼ cup buttermilk
- 2/3 cup whole-wheat panko or whole-wheat bread crumbs
- ½ cup grated Parmesan cheese (about 1½ ounces)
- ¾ teaspoon garlic powder, divided

- 1 cup canned low-sodium or no-salt-added crushed tomatoes

- 1 teaspoon dried oregano

- 6 (8-inch) whole-wheat tortillas, or whole-grain spinach wraps

- 1 cup fresh mozzarella cheese (about 4 ounces), sliced

- 1½ cups loosely packed fresh flat-leaf (Italian) parsley, chopped

DIRECTIONS:

1. Preheat the oven to 425°F. Line a large, rimmed baking sheet with aluminum foil. Place a wire rack on the aluminum foil, and spray the rack with nonstick cooking spray. Set aside.

2. Put the chicken breasts in a large, zip top plastic bag. With a rolling pin or meat mallet, pound the chicken so it is evenly flattened, about ¼ inch thick.

3. Slice the chicken into six portions. (It's fine if you have to place 2 smaller pieces together to form six equal portions.)

4. In a wide, shallow bowl, whisk together the egg and buttermilk. In another wide, shallow bowl, mix together the panko crumbs, Parmesan cheese, and ½ teaspoon of garlic powder.

5. Dip each chicken breast portion into the egg mixture and then into the Parmesan crumb mixture, pressing the crumbs into the chicken so they stick. Place the chicken on the prepared wire rack.

6. Bake the chicken for 15 to 18 minutes, or until the internal temperature of the chicken reads 165°F on a meat thermometer and any juices run clear.

7. Transfer the chicken to a cutting board, and slice each portion diagonally into ½-inch pieces.

8. In a small, microwave-safe bowl, mix together the tomatoes, oregano, and the remaining ¼ teaspoon of garlic powder.

9. Cover the bowl with a paper towel and microwave for about 1 minute on high, until very hot. Set aside.

10. Wrap the tortillas in a damp paper towel or dishcloth and microwave for 30 to 45 seconds on high, until warmed.

11. To assemble the wraps, divide the chicken slices evenly among the six tortillas and top with the cheese.

12. Spread 1 tablespoon of the warm tomato sauce over the cheese on each tortilla, and top each with about ¼ cup of parsley.

13. To wrap each tortilla, fold up the bottom of the tortilla, then fold one side over and fold the other side over the top. Serve the wraps immediately, with the remaining sauce for dipping.

NUTRITION: Calories: 373; Total Fat: 10g; Saturated Fat: 4g; Cholesterol: 95mg; Sodium: 591 mg; Total Carbohydrates: 33g; Fiber: 8g; Protein: 30g

85. Delicious Quinoa & Dried

Preparation Time: 10 minutes

Cooking Time: 17 minutes

Servings: 2

INGREDIENTS:

- 3 c. water
- ¼ c. cashew nut
- 8 dried apricots
- 4 dried figs

- 1 tsp. cinnamon
- Directions:
- In a pot, mix water and quinoa and
- Let simmer for 15 minutes, until the water evaporates.
- Chop dried fruit.
- When quinoa is cooked, stir in all other ingredients.
- Serve cold. Add milk, if desired.

NUTRITION: 44g Carbs, 7g Fat, 13g Protein, 285 Calories 65

86. Classic Apple Oats

Preparation Time: 10 minutes

Cooking Time: 15 minutes

Servings: 2

INGREDIENTS:

- ½ tsp. cinnamon
- ¼ tsp. ginger
- 2 apples make half-inch chunks
- ½ c. oats, steel cut
- 1½ c. water
- Maple syrup
- ¼ tsp. salt
- Clove
- ¼ tsp. nutmeg

DIRECTIONS:

1. Take Instant Pot and careful y arrange it over a clean, dry kitchen platform.

2. Turn on the appliance.

3. In the cooking pot area, add the water, oats, cinnamon, ginger, clove, nutmeg, apple, and salt. Stir the ingredients gently.

4. Close the pot lid and seal the valve to avoid any leakage. Find and press the "Manual" cooking setting and set cooking time to 5 minutes.

5. Allow the recipe ingredients to cook for the set time, and after that, the timer reads "zero."

6. Press "Cancel" and press "NPR" setting for natural pressure release. It takes 8-10 times for all inside pressure to release.

7. Open the pot and arrange the cooked recipe in serving plates.

8. Sweeten as needed with maple or agave syrup and serve immediately.

9. Top with some chopped nuts, optional.

NUTRITION: Calories: 232, Fat: 5.7 g, Carbs: 48.1 g, Protein: 5.2 g

87. Peach & Chia Seed

Preparation Time: 10 minutes

Cooking Time: 10 minutes

Servings: 2

INGREDIENTS:

- ½ oz. chia seeds
- 1 tbsp. pure maple syrup
- 1 c. coconut milk

- 1 tsp. ground cinnamon

- 3 diced peaches

- 2/3 c. granola

DIRECTIONS:

1. Find a small bowl and add the chia seeds, maple syrup, and coconut milk.

2. Stir well, then cover and pop into the fridge for at least one hour.

3. Find another bowl, add the peaches and sprinkle with the cinnamon. Pop to one side

4. When it's time to serve, take two glasses, and pour the chia mixture between the two.

5. Sprinkle the granola over the top, keeping a tiny amount to one side to use to decorate later.

6. Top with the peaches and top with the reserved granola and serve.

NUTRITION: Calories: 415, Protein: 13.9g, Carbs: 54.4g, Fat: 16.9g

88. Avocado Spread

Preparation Time: 10 minutes

Cooking Time: 1 minutes

Servings: 2

INGREDIENTS:

- 2 peeled and pitted avocados

- 1 tbsp. olive oil

- 1 tbsp. minced shallots

- 1 tbsp. lime juice
- 1 tbsp. heavy coconut cream
- Salt
- Black pepper
- 1 tbsp. chopped chives

DIRECTIONS:

1. In a blender, combine the avocado flesh with the oil, shallots, and the other ingredients except for the chopped chives.
2. Pulse well, divide into bowls, sprinkle the chives on top, and serve as a morning spread.

NUTRITION: Calories: 79, Fat: 0.4 g, Carbs: 15 g, Protein: 1.3 g

89. Almond Butter and Blueberry Smoothie

Preparation Time: 10 minutes

Cooking Time: 1 minutes

Servings: 2

INGREDIENTS:

- 1 c. almond milk
- 1 c. blueberries
- 4 ice cubes
- 1 scoop vanilla protein powder
- 1 tbsp. almond butter
- 1 tbsp. chia seeds

DIRECTIONS:

1. Use a blender to mix the almond butter, vanilla protein powder, chia seeds, almond milk, ice cubes and blueberries together until the consistency is smooth.

NUTRITION: Calories: 230, Carbs: 20 g, Fat: 8.1 g, Protein: 21.6 g

90. Salmon and Egg Muffins

Preparation Time: 10 minutes

Cooking Time: 15 minutes

Servings: 2

INGREDIENTS:

- 4 eggs
- 1/3 c. milk
- Salt and pepper
- 1½ oz. smoked salmon
- 1 tbsp. chopped chives
- Green onions, optional

DIRECTIONS:

2. Preheat the oven to 356 degrees Fahrenheit and grease 6 muffin tin holes with a small amount of olive oil.
3. Place the eggs, milk, and a pinch of salt and pepper into a small bowl and lightly beat to combine.
4. Divide the egg mixture between the 6 muffin holes, then divide the salmon between the muffins and place into each hole, gently pressing down to submerge in the egg mixture, chopped
5. Sprinkle each muffin with chopped chives and place in the oven for about 8-10 minutes or until just set.

6. Leave to cool for about 5 minutes before turning out and storing in an airtight container in the fridge.

NUTRITION: Calories: 93, Fat: 6g, Protein: 8g, Carbs: 1g

91. Nachos

Preparation Time: 5 Minutes

Cooking Time: 10 Minutes

Servings: 4

INGREDIENTS:

- 4-ounce restaurant-style corn tortilla chips
- 1 medium green onion, thinly sliced (about 1 tbsp.)
- 1 (4 ounces) package finely crumbled feta cheese
- 1 finely chopped and drained plum tomato
- 2 tbsp Sun-dried tomatoes in oil, finely chopped
- 2 tbsp Kalamata olives

DIRECTIONS:

1. Mix an onion, plum tomato, oil, sun-dried tomatoes, and olives in a small bowl.

2. Arrange the tortillas chips on a microwavable plate in a single layer topped evenly with cheese—microwave on high for one minute.

3. Rotate the plate half turn and continue microwaving until the cheese is bubbly. Spread the tomato mixture over the chips and cheese and enjoy.

NUTRITION: Calories: 140 Carbs: 19g Fat: 7g Protein: 2g

DESSERT RECIPES

92. Mini Orange Tarts

Preparation Time: 45 minutes

Cooking Time: 0 minutes

Servings: 2

INGREDIENTS

- 1 cup coconut flour
- 1/2 cup almond flour
- A pinch of grated nutmeg
- A pinch of sea salt
- 1/4 teaspoon ground cloves
- 1/4 teaspoon ground anise
- 1 cup brown sugar
- 6 eggs
- 2 cups heavy cream
- 2 oranges, peeled and sliced

DIRECTIONS

1. Begin by preheating your oven to 350 degrees F.
2. Thoroughly combine the flour with spices. Stir in the sugar, eggs, and heavy cream. Mix again to combine well.
3. Divide the batter into six lightly greased ramekins.

4. Top with the oranges and bake in the preheated oven for about 40 minutes until the clafoutis is just set. Bon appétit!

NUTRITION: Calories: 398; Fat: 28.5g; Carbs: 24.9g; Protein: 11.9g

93. Traditional Kalo Prama

Preparation Time: 45 minutes

Cooking Time: 0 minutes

Servings: 2

INGREDIENTS

- 2 large eggs
- 1/2 cup Greek yogurt
- 1/2 cup coconut oil
- 1/2 cup sugar
- 8 ounces semolina
- 1 teaspoon baking soda
- 2 tablespoons walnuts, chopped
- 1/4 teaspoon ground nutmeg
- 1/4 teaspoon ground anise
- 1/2 teaspoon ground cinnamon
- 1 cup water
- 1 ½ cups caster sugar
- 1 teaspoon lemon zest
- 1 teaspoon lemon juice

DIRECTIONS

1. Thoroughly combine the eggs, yogurt, coconut oil, and sugar. Add in the semolina, baking soda, walnuts, nutmeg, anise, and cinnamon.
2. Let it rest for 1 ½ hour.
3. Bake in the preheated oven at 350 degrees F for approximately 40 minutes or until a tester inserted in the center of the cake comes out dry and clean.
4. Transfer to a wire rack to cool completely before slicing.
5. Meanwhile, bring the water and caster sugar to a full boil; add in the lemon zest and lemon juice, and turn the heat to a simmer; let it simmer for about 8 minutes or until the sauce has thickened slightly.
6. Cut the cake into diamonds and pour the syrup over the top; allow it to soak for about 2 hours. Bon appétit!

NUTRITION: Calories: 478; Fat: 22.5g; Carbs: 62.4g; Protein: 8.2g

94. Turkish-Style Chocolate Halva

Preparation Time: 20 minutes

Cooking Time: 0 minutes

Servings: 2

INGREDIENTS

- 1/2 cup water
- 2 cups sugar
- 2 cups tahini
- 1/4 teaspoon cardamom
- 1/4 teaspoon cinnamon

- A pinch of sea salt
- 6 ounces dark chocolate, broken into chunks

DIRECTIONS

1. Bring the water to a full boil in a small saucepan. Add in the sugar and stir. Let it cook, stirring occasionally, until a candy thermometer registers 250 degrees F. Heat off.

2. Stir in the tahini. Continue to stir with a wooden spoon just until halva comes together in a smooth mass; do not overmix your halva.

3. Add in the cardamom, cinnamon, and salt; stir again to combine well. Now, scrape your halva into a parchment-lined square pan.

4. Microwave the chocolate until melted; pour the melted chocolate over your halva and smooth the top.

5. Let it cool to room temperature; cover tightly with a plastic wrap and place in your refrigerator for at least 2 hours. Bon appétit!

NUTRITION: Calories: 388; Fat: 27.5g; Carbs: 31.6g; Protein: 7.9g

95. Rice Pudding with Dried Figs

Preparation Time: 45 minutes

Cooking Time: 0 minutes

Servings: 2

INGREDIENTS

- 3 cups milk
- 1 cup water
- 2 tablespoons sugar
- 1/3 cup white rice, rinsed

- 1 tablespoon honey
- 4 dried figs, chopped
- 1/2 teaspoon cinnamon
- 1/2 teaspoon rose water

DIRECTIONS

1. In a deep saucepan, bring the milk, water and sugar to a boil until the sugar has dissolved.
2. Stir in the rice, honey, figs, raisins, cinnamon, and turn the heat to a simmer; let it simmer for about 40 minutes, stirring periodically to prevent your pudding from sticking.
3. Afterwards, stir in the rose water. Divide the pudding between individual bowls and serve. Bon appétit!

NUTRITION: Calories: 228; Fat: 6.1g; Carbs: 35.1g; Protein: 7.1g

96. Fruit Kabobs with Yogurt Deep

Preparation Time: 10 minutes

Cooking Time: 0 minutes

Servings: 2

INGREDIENTS

- 8 clementine orange segments
- 8 medium-sized strawberries
- 8 pineapple cubes
- 8 seedless grapes
- 1/2 cup Greek-style yogurt
- 1/2 teaspoon vanilla extract

- 2 tablespoons honey

DIRECTIONS

1. Thread the fruits onto 4 skewers.

2. In a mixing dish, thoroughly combine the yogurt, vanilla, and honey.

3. Serve alongside your fruit kabobs for dipping. Bon appétit!

NUTRITION: Calories: 98; Fat: 0.2g; Carbs: 20.7g; Protein: 2.8g

97. No-Bake Chocolate Squares

Preparation Time: 10 minutes

Cooking Time: 0 minutes

Servings: 2

INGREDIENTS

- 8 ounces bittersweet chocolate

- 1 cup tahini paste

- 1/4 cup almonds, chopped

- 1/4 cup walnuts, chopped

DIRECTIONS

1. Microwave the chocolate for about 30 seconds or until melted. Stir in the tahini, almonds, and walnuts.

2. Spread the batter into a parchment-lined baking pan. Place in your refrigerator until set, for about 3 hours.

3. Cut into squares and serve well-chilled. Bon appétit!

NUTRITION: Calories: 198; Fat: 13g; Carbs: 17.3g; Protein: 4.6g

98. Greek Parfait with Mixed Berries

Preparation Time: 10 minutes

Cooking Time: 0 minutes

Servings: 2

INGREDIENTS

- 2 cups Greek yogurt
- 2 cups mixed berries
- 1/2 cup granola

DIRECTIONS

1. Alternate layers of mixed berries, granola, and yogurt until two dessert bowls are filled completely.
2. Cover and place in your refrigerator until you're ready to serve. Bon appétit!

NUTRITION: Calories: 238; Fat: 16.7g; Carbs: 53g; Protein: 21.6g

99. Greek-Style Chocolate Semifreddo

Preparation Time: 15 minutes

Cooking Time: 0 minutes

Servings: 2

INGREDIENTS

- 3 ounces dark chocolate, broken into chunks
- 1 teaspoon vanilla extract
- A pinch of grated nutmeg
- A pinch of sea salt
- 1 cup heavy cream, divided

- 2 egg whites, at room temperature

- 1/2 cup caster sugar

- 4 tablespoons water

- 1/2 cup plain Greek yogurt

- 1 tablespoon brandy

- 2 tablespoons dark chocolate curls, to decorate

DIRECTIONS

1. In a glass bowl, thoroughly combine the chocolate, vanilla, nutmeg, and sea salt.

2. In a small saucepan, bring the cream to a simmer. Pour the hot cream over the chocolate mixture and stir until everything is well incorporated.

3. Place in your refrigerator for about 1 hour.

4. Now, mix the egg whites on high speed until soft peaks form.

5. Dissolve the sugar in water over medium-low heat until a candy thermometer registers 250 degrees F or until the syrup has thickened.

6. Now, pour the syrup into the beaten egg whites and continue to beat until glossy. Fold in the chilled chocolate mixture, Greek yogurt, and brandy; mix again until everything is well combined.

7. Freeze your dessert for at least 3 hours. Then, let it sit at room temperature for about 15 minutes before slicing and serving. Top with the chocolate curls. Bon appétit!

NUTRITION: Calories: 517; Fat: 27.7g; Carbs: 61g; Protein: 6.8g

100. Traditional Italian Cake with Almonds

Preparation Time: 45 minutes

Cooking Time: 0 minutes

Servings: 2

INGREDIENTS

- 4 ripe peaches, peeled, pitted, and sliced
- 1 tablespoon fresh lemon juice
- 2 ¼ cups all-purpose flour
- 1 teaspoon baking soda
- 1/2 teaspoon baking powder
- A pinch of grated nutmeg
- A pinch of sea salt
- 1/2 teaspoon ground cloves
- 1/2 teaspoon ground cinnamon
- 1/2 cup olive oil
- 1 1/3 cups sugar
- 3 eggs, at room temperature
- 1 cup Greek yogurt
- 1 teaspoon pure vanilla extract
- 1/2 cup almonds, chopped

DIRECTIONS

1. Begin by preheating your oven to 350 degrees F. Toss the peaches with lemon juice and set them aside.

2. Then, thoroughly combine the dry ingredients.

3. Then, beat the olive oil and sugar using your mixer at low speed.

4. Gradually fold in the eggs, one at a time, and continue to mix for a few minutes more until it has thickened. Add in the yogurt and vanilla, and mix again.

5. Add the wet mixture to the dry ingredients and stir until you get a thick batter. Fold in the almonds and stir to combine well.

6. Spoon the batter into a parchment-lined baking pan and level the top using a wooden spoon.

7. Bake in the preheated oven for about 40 minutes or until a tester comes out dry and clean. Let it cool on a wire rack before slicing and serving. Bon appétit!

NUTRITION: Calories: 407; Fat: 14.7g; Carbs: 61.4g; Protein: 6.6g

101. Stuffed Dried Figs

Preparation Time: 20 Minutes

Cooking Time: 0 Minutes

Servings: 4

INGREDIENTS:

- 12 dried figs
- 2 Tbsps. thyme honey
- 2 Tbsps. sesame seeds
- 24 walnut halves

DIRECTIONS:

1. Cut off the tough stalk ends of the figs.
2. Slice open each fig.
3. Stuff the fig openings with two walnut halves and close

4. Arrange the figs on a plate, drizzle with honey, and sprinkle the sesame seeds on it.

5. Serve.

NUTRITION: Calories: 110kcal Carbs: 26 Fat: 3g, Protein: 1g

CONCLUSION

Thank you for reaching the end of this book.

As we close this book, I want to share some important things about Mediterranean Diet that will really help you.

When starting anything new, mistakes are unavoidable. In this chapter, I am going to give you a quick rundown of some of the mistakes I made when I first started eating the Mediterranean way, as well as share some slipups friends and family members had.

Mistake 1: Portion Control

I know I've been going on and on about moderation. I will, unfortunately, have to talk about it some more under the guise of portion control. Managing how much you eat is particularly important if you're trying to lose weight, but it is also a factor if you want to maintain your weight and, with it, your health.

It's not about controlling the number of vegetables you're eating. We've established that you will instinctively eat until you're full since veggies are high in fiber and, therefore, very filling.

You have to regulate everything else on your plate. Nuts and olive oil are the main culprits in eating too many calories without even realizing it. A recommended daily serving of nuts is one to two handfuls. Olive oil should be limited to two tablespoons per dish.

Mistake 2: Carb Overload

Although the Mediterranean Diet includes grains and cereals, including the oh-so-addicting bread and pasta varieties, it doesn't mean you should overeat. It is healthier to limit your carbohydrate intake, especially refined carbs, for all the reasons I mentioned earlier while discussing the Mediterranean food pyramid.

To motivate my reasoning even further, consider the fact that we are more sedentary than the people who traditionally worked the farms and went fishing. We drive and don't walk, and we take the escalator instead of using the stairs. The examples are endless.

This lower level of activity means we burn fewer calories than our ancestors, but we still want to eat more while doing less. No wonder so many people are overweight!

Mistake 3: Not Eating Enough Fish

You won't reap the heart- and brain-boosting health benefits of fish and seafood if you don't eat enough of it. Aim for three times a week, and you'll get all the omega-3 fatty acids your brain and body need.

If you're a vegetarian or you dislike seafood, don't worry, just supplement with fish and seaweed oil.

Mistake 4: Eating the Wrong Dairy

Not all cheese is good for you. Pasteurized cheese, for example, isn't as nutrient-rich and doesn't contain as many probiotics as feta, mozzarella, Camembert. This also applies to yogurt. If you choose to buy those that are artificially flavored and packed full of sugar, you won't be doing your gut any favors. However, if you select plain Greek yogurt or, better yet, kefir, and flavor it yourself with fruit, nuts, and even some honey, your insides will do a happy dance.

Mistake 5: Banishing the Beans

Beans should be part of a healthy foundation of the Mediterranean meal plan. Some people prefer to leave this superfood off their plates because it takes longer to prepare than other food, and beans give some people gas. Considering that beans are oxidation fighters and helpful in regulating blood sugar, I suggest you put aside any objections you have against eating them.

Mistake 6: Thinking Wine is Water

It can be tempting to drink more wine than you're allowed. Yes, red wine does have health benefits as mentioned in the previous chapter. But it can't nor should it replace water.

First off, wine is not going to quench your thirst. It will actually make you thirstier. Also, the advantages of drinking water should not be overlooked. It's good for your kidneys and all other organs too, come to think of it. It helps your digestive system run smoothly. And my favorite perk from drinking enough water – soft, glowing skin.

Mistake 7: Using Extra-Virgin Olive Oil at a High Heat

When extra-virgin olive oil reaches 400 degrees Fahrenheit, it starts losing all the stuff that makes it good, as well as its flavor. Even more concerning, the oil will become pro-inflammatory due to the oxidation that takes place through heat damage. As you can see, overheating extra-virgin olive oil will not only damage your health but your pocketbook too. Who wants to eat olive oil with no taste?

Mistake 8: Not Obeying the 10 Commandments

It's not as serious as it sounds, I promise. But the 10 commandments perfectly sum up what the Mediterranean Diet and lifestyle is all about. And, if you follow them diligently, you're set to gain a healthy body and a longer life.

Don't worry if you wander off the path now and again. You won't be condemned to a sickly life spent in an out of shape body. Just get back to following the Mediterranean Diet and living the lifestyle, and you'll be A-Okay.

The ten commandments of the Mediterranean Diet and lifestyle are:

1. Fill your plate with an abundance of fresh, non-processed food.

2. Do not let any saturated fat, trans fat, sodium, or refined sugar cross your lips.

3. Don't use margarine or butter; in its place use olive oil or trans-fat-free vegetable spread.

4. Eat your fill of vegetables but limit the portions of other foods.

5. Drink enough water.

6. Don't drink too much red wine.

7. Get your heart rate up for at least 30 minutes a day.

8. Don't smoke.

9. Unwind and relax, specifically after eating.

10. Laugh a lot, smile, and enjoy life.

Thank you and Good luck.

CPSIA information can be obtained
at www.ICGtesting.com
Printed in the USA
LVHW060935130221
679241LV00001B/25

9 781801 651790